The Survive and Thrive Guide to
COMPUTER VALIDATION

■■■

Teri Stokes, Ph.D.

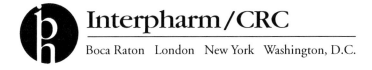

Interpharm/CRC

Boca Raton   London   New York   Washington, D.C.

Library of Congress Cataloging-in-Publication Data

Stokes, Teri
    The survive and thrive guide to computer validation / Teri Stokes.
        p. cm. .
    Includes bibliographical references and index.
    ISBN 1-57491-067-1
        1. Computer software—Validation. 2.Computer sofware—Quality control.
    3. Electronic digital computers—evaluation.   I. Title
    QA76.76. V47S76   1998
    005.1´4—dc21   98-18089

This book contains information obtained from authentic and highly regarded sources. Reprinted material is quoted with permission, and sources are indicated. A wide variety of references are listed. Reasonable efforts have been made to publish reliable data and information, but the author and the publisher cannot assume responsibility for the validity of all materials or for the consequences of their use.

Neither this book nor any part may be reproduced or transmitted in any form or by any means, electronic or mechanical, including photocopying, microfilming, and recording, or by any information storage or retrieval system, without prior permission in writing from the publisher.

The consent of CRC Press LLC does not extend to copying for general distribution, for promotion, for creating new works, or for resale. Specific permission must be obtained in writing from CRC Press LLC for such copying.

Direct all inquiries to CRC Press LLC, 2000 N.W. Corporate Blvd., Boca Raton, Florida 33431.

Trademark Notice: Product or corporate names may be trademarks or registered trademarks, and are used only for identification and explanation, without intent to infringe.

Visit the CRC Press Web site at www.crcpress.com

© 1998 by CRC Press LLC
Interpharm is an imprint of CRC Press

No claim to original U.S. Government works
International Standard Book Number 1-57491-067-1
Library of Congress Card Number 98-18089
Printed in the United States of America 1 2 3 4 5 6 7 8 9 0
Printed on acid-free paper

Contents

Preface	**xiii**
Global Perspectives	**xv**

1. Introduction: Team and System Concepts for Computer Validation — 1

I. System Sponsor's Summary	1
What Is Computer Validation?	*1*
The System Sponsor	*2*
II. System Owner and System Team Discussion	3
The System Owner	*3*
The System Validation Team or System Team	*3*
System Concepts	*5*
Quality Concepts for Computerized Systems	*9*
III. Conclusion	12
Why Validate?	*12*

2. Managing System Life Cycles — 15

I. System Sponsor's Summary	15
Return on Investment	*15*
System Life Cycle and Owner Selection	*15*
II. System Owner and System Team Discussion	16
Phase 1. System Idea	*17*
Phase 2. System Plan	*20*

iv   The Survive and Thrive Guide to Computer Validation

Phase 3. Design	*24*
Phase 4. Build	*25*
Phase 5. Test	*26*
Phase 6. Commission	*27*
Phase 7. Operate	*29*
Phase 8. Maintain	*30*
Phase 9. Retire	*31*
III. Conclusion	34
Validation Is a Lifetime Process for a Regulated System	*34*
Custom-Built Systems Increase the Owner's Life Cycle Work	*34*

3. The Supplier's Verification Package   37

I. System Sponsor's Summary	37
II. System Owner and System Team Discussion	39
The Purchaser's Representative	*40*
The Supplier's Representative	*41*
Supplier's Verification Plan	*42*
Engineering SOPs	*43*
Configuration Management Logs	*45*
System Design Description (SDD)	*46*
Development Documentation	*47*
Quality Plan and Supplier Self-Audit Reports	*48*
Verification Testing	*49*
System Documents	*50*
Training Materials and Support Plan	*51*
Test Plan(s)	*51*
Test Scripts, Test Data, and Result Logs	*52*
Test Summary Report	*54*
Verification Summary Report	*54*
III. Conclusion	55
System Quality Must Be Planned, Built-in, and Documented, *Not Discovered*	*55*

4. The Owner's Validation Package   57

I. System Sponsor's Summary   57

II. System Owner and System Team Discussion   59

Owner's Validation Plan   60

Validation Testing   63

Validation Test Plan(s)   64

Test Scripts, Test Data, and Result Logs   66

Test Summary Report   69

Commission Phase Testing-Acceptance, IQ, OQ, PQ   70

Operation Phase Validation   71

System Standard Operating Procedures (SOPs)   72

System Management Logs   74

Platform and Support Plan and Contracts   74

Audit Reports   74

Ongoing Quality Control Testing and Repeat Validation Testing   75

System and User Documents and Training Program   75

Validation Summary Report   76

III. Conclusion   77

A Standard System Package Supports System Reliability and Inspectability   77

5. The Retrospective Evaluation Package   79

I. System Sponsor's Summary   79

II. System Owner and System Team Discussion   81

The Evaluation Plan   82

Timeline and History   83

System SOPs and System Logs   86

System and User Documents   91

Audit Reports and Quality Control Records   93

Evaluation Testing of a Legacy System   94

Evaluation Summary Report   97

vi   The Survive and Thrive Guide to Computer Validation

III. Conclusion	98
Legacy Systems Need Validation Work to Perform Regulated Tasks Today	*98*
6. The Systems Quality Assurance Plan (SQAP)	**101**
I. System Sponsor's Summary	101
A Logical Approach to Multiple Systems	*101*
II. System Owner and System Team Discussion	102
SQAPs for Control of a Multiple Systems Environment	*102*
SQAP Outline	*104*
Developing an SQAP	*104*
Purpose	*107*
Scope	*107*
Reference Documents	*109*
Management	*109*
Documentation	*111*
Standards, Practices, and Metrics	*111*
Reviews, Audits, and Inspections	*114*
System Testing	*115*
Problem Reporting and Corrective Action	*116*
Code and Media Control	*118*
Supplier Control	*120*
Records Collection, Maintenance, and Retention	*120*
Training	*121*
Risk Management	*122*
Approvals	*122*
Appendices	*123*
III. Conclusion	123
An SQAP Focuses System Team Efforts to Save Time and Prioritize Systems	*123*

Contents   vii

7. Computer Validation Policy   125

I. System Sponsor's Summary   125

Policy—The Role for Senior Management in Computer Validation   *125*

II. System Owner and System Team Discussion   127

Developing a Computer Validation Policy   *128*

Content for a Computer Validation Policy   *130*

Policy Requirements Models   *132*

III. Conclusion   140

Implementing a C.V. Policy Brings Good Business Benefits   *140*

8. International Regulations and Directives   143

I. System Sponsor's Summary   143

Regulatory Timeline   *143*

II. System Owner and System Team Discussion   145

EU GMP Guide Annex 11: Computerized Systems   *145*

OECD GLP Consensus: Application of GLP Principles to Computerized Systems   *147*

FDA—Electronic Records; Electronic Signatures; Final Rule   *149*

FDA's Blue Book for cGMP Systems   *152*

FDA Computerized Medical Device GMP   *154*

Japan's Ministry of Health and Welfare (MHW)—GMP Guideline   *155*

ICH Good Clinical Practice (GCP) Directive   *159*

ICH Guideline on Statistical Principles for Clinical Trials   *161*

III. Conclusion   162

World Authorities Are Increasing C.V. Directives for GXP Systems   *162*

9. Survive and Thrive with Reviews, Audits, and Inspections   165

I. System Sponsor's Summary   165

Audit Perspectives and ROI—What They See Is What You've Got   *165*

II. System Owner and System Team Discussion   168

viii   The Survive and Thrive Guide to Computer Validation

Standards for Examination Exercises	*169*
Walk-Through Review Process	*172*
Walk-Through Preparation and Activity	*172*
Walk-Through Report and Gap Analysis	*174*
Benefits of a Walk-Through and Gap Analysis	*175*
SOP for Systems Audit or Inspection	*176*
Follow-up Actions to Audits and Inspections	*179*
Regulatory Consequences for Inspection Issues	*180*
III. Conclusion	181
Pride in System Performance	*181*

10. Laboratory Systems — 183

I. System Sponsor's Summary	183
Automation and LIMS-Good Automated Laboratory Practice (GALP)	*184*
II. System Owner and System Team Discussion	186
Step 1: Walk-Through Review, Systems Inventory, and Gap Analysis	*186*
Step 2: SQAP Development and Policy Statement	*187*
Step 3: Standard Operating Procedures	*187*
Step 4: Assign Teams and Develop System Packages	*189*
Step 5: Use a Standard Laboratory Data Handling Model	*190*
Step 6: Establish Instrument Automation Logbooks	*192*
Step 7: Document Legacy Automation Systems	*193*
Step 8: Plan for Electronic Records Retention and System Retirement	*195*
Step 9: Practice for Audits and Inspections	*196*
III. Conclusion	198
Simple Definition and Defined Approach	*198*

11. Clinical Research Systems — 199

I. System Sponsor's Summary	199
System Categories—Trial Sponsor and Nonsponsor, GCP and Non-GCP	*201*
II. System Owner and System Team Discussion	203

Step 1: Identify and Validate General Systems at
Trial Sponsor Location(s) — 204

Step 2: Identify and Validate Custom-Built or Specialty
GCP Clinical Systems — 204

Step 3: Identify Protocol-specific Systems — 205

Step 4: Prepare e-Quality Action Sections for Medical Monitoring
and Data Management Plans — 207

Step 5: Develop an Electronic Data Quality Plan (EDQ Plan)
for the Protocol — 208

Step 6: Develop Practical Field Action Guidelines — 209

III. Conclusion — 214

Identify GCP Study Systems and Plan a Pragmatic Approach — 214

12. Manufacturing Systems — 217

I. System Sponsor's Summary — 217

GMP Status and Validation Priority — 217

II. System Owner and System Team Discussion — 219

Step 1: Conduct a Walk-Through of the Facility or
New Product Life Cycle — 221

Step 2: Develop a C.V. Policy Statement and an SQAP — 223

Step 3: Standard Operating Procedures — 224

Step 4: Assign System Teams and Develop Standard
Validation Packages — 226

Step 5: Train All Site Personnel to GMP System Validation Concepts — 227

Step 6: Take a Product Life Cycle Approach to Large and
Legacy Systems — 228

Step 7: Plan for Electronic Records Retention and
Electronic Signature Use — 230

Step 8: Prepare for Audits and Inspections — 232

III. Conclusion — 233

Product "X" Life Cycle Approach and SEQ Priority — 233

x   **The Survive and Thrive Guide to Computer Validation**

13. GMP References (EU and Japan), Electronic Records and Electronic Signatures (US)   **235**

I. Introduction   235

European Union (EU)   235

Ministry of Health and Welfare (MHW) Japan   235

U.S. Food and Drug Administration   236

II. EU GMP GUIDE—Annex 11 and Excerpts of Chapters 4 & 7   237

Annex 11—Pages 139-142   237

EU GMP Guide Chapter 4—Documentation   239

EU GMP Guide Chapter 7—Contract Manufacture and Analysis   240

III. MHW—Japan—Guideline on Control of Computerized Systems in Drug Manufacturing   243

Part 1: Objectives   243

Part 2: Scope of Application   243

Part 3: Development of the System   244

Part 4: Operation Control   248

Part 5: Documentation (Including Plan, Procedures, and Others)   252

Part 6: Date of Enforcement   252

IV. U.S. FDA 21 CFR Part 11 Electronic Records; Electronic Signatures; Final Rule—Excerpts   253

Subpart B: Electronic Records   253

Subpart C: Electronic Signatures   255

14. OECD GLP and U.S. EPA GALP Excerpts   **257**

Introduction—Document Contacts   257

Organization for Economic Cooperation and Development (OECD)   257

U.S. Environmental Protection Agency (EPA)   257

GLP Consensus Document: The Application of the Principles of GLP to Computerized Systems—OECD, Paris, 1995   258

Scope   258

Approach   258

The Application of the GLP Principles to Computerized Systems   259

EPA 2185—Good Automated Laboratory Practices (GALP)	270
Scope	*270*
8. Good Automated Laboratory Practices	270

15. ICH and FDA Guidelines for GCP Systems—Excerpts — 277

Introduction-Document Sources	277
U.S. Food and Drug Administration	*277*
ICH GCP—Computer Relevant Excerpts	279
ICH Topic E6—Guideline for Good Clinical Practice—EMEA—for Trials Starting After January 17, 1997	*279*
FDA Draft Guidance—Computerized Systems Used in Clinical Trials	285

Index — 297

Preface

Welcome to the adventure of computer validation! Basing your efforts on a standards-based approach and using your uncommon "common sense" gained from experience with your regulated systems, you too can survive the validation experience. In fact, getting your validation house in order will give your business a boost by ensuring system reliability and data integrity so that the business thrives on the benefits of its strategic systems performing as intended.

Today's world depends on computerized systems performing their intended functions in a controlled, reliable manner. This book describes an approach to computer validation that is based on practical project experience in many pharmaceutical, biotech, and software companies around the world. Its recommendations address two basic perspectives:

- To survive as a company in a regulated industry, it is essential to validate strategic systems to be sure they work correctly and can pass inspections.

- To validate and still thrive as a business, it is necessary to develop validation practices that fit into an organization's culture and become integrated into the normal workflow of regulated activities.

Just like validating a system, writing a book is a team effort, and I would like to thank my husband Peter Rice Yensen for nursing me through the three months of post-surgery convalescence during which I wrote this manuscript. Many thanks to H. Matsui-san for English versions of the MHW regulations and to Amy Davis and Jane Steinmann for editing and publishing support at Interpharm Press.

Special appreciation goes to Jane Ganter, editor of *Applied Clinical Trials*, for starting me down the trail to this book by having me write a six-part series of Technical Update articles on GCP systems. Writing the series forced me to organize my thinking about the discipline of computer validation. The title of the book and much of the content in Chapter 9, on reviews, audits, and inspections, come from

xiv   The Survive and Thrive Guide to Computer Validation

the last article in the series—"A Survive and Thrive Approach to Audits and Inspections," *Applied Clinical Trials*, August 1997.

Since the regulations for computer validation are international in scope and the regulated industries operate on a global basis, I thought it important to have prefatory perspectives about validation by other professionals of international repute from North America, Europe, and Japan. It is an honor to have three world experts give their views in the "Global Perspectives" section that follows, and I would like to thank my colleagues Dr. Richard Chamberlain, Dr. Bob McDowall, and Yasuo Bando-san for sharing their professional views on computer validation.

With warm wishes for your every success,

Teri Stokes, Ph.D.
Director
GXP International
May 1998

■ Global Perspectives

NORTH AMERICA—R. L. Chamberlain, Ph.D.

Dr. Richard Chamberlain is President of Executive Consultant Services, Inc., providing software validation solutions for pharmaceutical and medical device clients in North America and abroad. With over 25 years of industry experience at Abbott Laboratories and Medical Development Systems, Dr. Chamberlain was active in establishing the Computer Systems Validation Committee of the Pharmaceutical Research and Manufacturers of America (PhRMA). He also is author of several books on the subject of computer systems validation and systems auditing.

The current interest in computer systems validation really began in 1983 when the U.S. Food and Drug Administration (FDA) issued the now well-known "Blue Book": *A Guide to Inspection of Computerized Drug Processing Systems*. Since then, a variety of books, guidelines, regulations, and other documents has attempted to clarify the requirements for computer systems validation. In this book, Teri Stokes has presented several very important aspects of computer systems validation that need to be understood regardless of the type or complexity of the system.

Computer Systems Validation As a Process

The concepts surrounding process validation are well known and well documented. Computer systems validation is process validation. The process being validated is the process used to develop, support, and maintain a computer system. Without a well-defined process for developing computer systems, it is impossible to talk about validation. By "well defined" we mean having written standard operating procedures (SOPs) that define the tasks involved in the process, the clear assignment of responsibilities, and tangible deliverables. The

xvi The Survive and Thrive Guide to Computer Validation

outline of this process is referred to as a system development life cycle (SDLC), and the various forms of this outline have been well known for over 40 years. There certainly is no need to reinvent it. Teri uses this concept as the basis for most of the chapters in her book.

Quality Assurance and Quality Control Are Part of the Process

I tend to think of Quality Control as those checks done by the people doing the work while they are doing it. Quality Assurance involves those checks done by an independent group. They may be the same checks in both cases. QC and QA are concepts popularized by W. E. Deming in Japan following World War II, and they are credited with placing Japan in its current successful economy. The notions of Total Quality Management (TQM), ISO, and the current GMPs use QC and QA as their cornerstone. Teri is able to show the involvement of QC and QA in the systems development process in a logical and positive way.

Regardless of the System, the Same Basic Process Applies

The various types of systems you encounter can all use the same basic model or SDLC. Whether the system is developed in house, purchased, configured, off-the-shelf (OTS), or a legacy program, the same model can be used. It may be that some of the phases of the SDLC are not needed or are done by the vendor. In any case one has to consider the complete model. Throughout this book, Teri makes the point very well that the same model applies.

Testing Must Be Against Something

Any book on testing will say that a good test case has at least three components:

1. The input to the test
2. The output from the test
3. The EXPECTED output from the test

Many people to omit the third component. However, you cannot simply test— you must test against something. It is not good enough for the testers simply to say, "here is the input; there is the output; it passes." They must say, "here is the input; there is the output; *this is what the output was supposed to be*; it passes." Where does the expected output come from? It comes from the requirements, design, and other specifications. Without these documents, it is impossible to test a system. Teri makes this lesson clear in every chapter where testing is discussed.

Documentation Is Where It's At

The process must produce documentation. I like to relate the story of my Ph.D. thesis and documentation. When I started my Ph.D., I was fortunate to work under the relatively well-known statistician and geneticist, Oscar Kempthorne. At the time, he had a contemporary who claimed to have a computer program that would analyze any experimental design, no matter how complex. Design of experiments was one of Kempthorne's specialties, and he was suspicious of the claim. For my thesis, he presented me with a theorem that would prove his counterpart wrong.

I worked on that theorem for two years and was unable to prove it. Then one day, the light went on, and I said to myself, "Suppose Kempthorne's wrong, and the theorem is not true?" It took me about an hour to develop a counterexample to show that the theorem was false. Fortunately for me, I had done enough research over the two years that I could see how the theorem should be stated so that it was true and yet also show that his counterpart was wrong. I spent a week writing this up and presented it to Kempthorne. He looked intently at it, leaned back in his chair, and said, "You know, Dick, the written word is very unreliable." Then he leaned forward until he was only four inches from my face and added, "but it is the only thing we have." He was telling me to write it up, but he also was right when he said, "it is the only thing we have." Without information in writing, or some other semipermanent form, we have nothing!

Unless things are written down, the process does not exist, and the system is incomplete. Without proper documentation, the system cannot be used or maintained properly, and it certainly cannot be validated. Teri does an excellent job of making the point that regardless of the variation of the SDLC you use, it must produce documentation.

This book is unique in the way it covers the breadth of computer systems validation for a variety of readers. Users, information technology professionals, and quality assurance staff can all benefit from its contents.

Richard L. Chamberlain, Ph.D.
President
Executive Consultant Services, Inc.
May 1998

EUROPE—R. D. McDowall, Ph.D.

Dr. R. D. McDowall is Principal of McDowall Consulting and a NAMAS (National Accreditation of Measurement and Sampling) assessor specializing in separation sciences and computer validation for chromatography data systems, LIMS, and laboratory automation. With 15 years of industry experience at SmithKline French Research Laboratories and Wellcome Research Laboratories, Dr. McDowall consults to the healthcare industry across Europe for the validation of laboratory and clinical systems. He is leader of the annual course for Practical Computer Validation provided by the Royal Pharmaceutical Society of Great Britain.

FDA inspections of computerised systems in U.S. pharmaceutical companies from 1983 onwards had an impact on European companies that were subject to FDA inspection. Regulations and initiatives related to validation of computerised systems in Europe followed from this. To give an overview of the European perspective on computerised system validation, I want to look at each of the affected areas in turn, with respect to the pharmaceutical industry first.

Good Laboratory Practice (GLP)

Initiatives to provide guidelines on the application of GLP principles to computerised systems started in the United Kingdom in 1989 with the introduction of *Advisory Leaflet Number 1* by the Department of Health [1]. This was the first time that the UK authorities had put pen to paper about computerised systems and GLP. Its emphasis was very much on what an inspector was expecting to see. However, it had one minor problem: It did not actually mention the word *validation* anywhere in the document. *Advisory 1* was updated in 1995 [2], making the text clearer but maintaining the emphasis on testing rather than validation (although *validation* was used once in the context of data migration to a replacement system).

In parallel with the update of the UK leaflet, the Organisation of Economic Co-operation and Development (OECD), based in Paris, produced a consensus document that interpreted GLP principles for computerised systems [3]. This document, similar to all international GLP regulations, emphasizes inspection more than the development of the system. However, it is an advance as it specifically discusses vendor audits.

Good Manufacturing Practice (GMP)

European Directive 91/356/EEC [4] led to the writing of GMP Annex 11 for computerised systems in the 1993 Orange Guide [5]. This annex presents guiding principles for the use of computerised systems, followed by 19 criteria that systems should meet. The document provides a philosophy of system development and operation and, in my view, is probably the best overall regulatory guideline. The criteria leave room for individual interpretation and flexibility for different types of system. To help companies, the German APV have produced an interpretation of these guidelines [6]. The EU GMP guidelines were updated in 1997 [7], but Annex 11 was not modified—missing an opportunity to incorporate the APV interpretation.

Similar to the actions by the Pharmaceutical Manufacturing Association (PMA) and Parenteral Drug Association (PDA) in the United States, industry initiatives in Europe have attempted to move the emphasis from regulations to a voluntary code of practice for computer validation. Started in the United Kingdom, the UK Pharmaceutical Industry Computerised System Validation Forum (UKPICSV) was the original vehicle for developing a code of practice between industry and suppliers. The draft version of the guide was issued in March 1994 and finalised later that year. The second version of the Good Automated Manufacturing Practice (GAMP) Guide was released in May 1996 [8]. Available in both hard copy and electronic copy, GAMP is now sponsored by the International Society for Pharmaceutical Engineering (ISPE).

The GAMP Guide contains 10 main chapters overviewing the validation of systems, followed by 28 appendices covering the system life cycle, from a guide for a user requirements specification to the APV interpretation of the GMP guidelines discussed above. The electronic version of the GAMP Guide is a hypertext document which is very useful for searching for items. The third version of the GAMP Guide will be released in 1998. Evidence of the usefulness of the Guide is that it has been taken up as the corporate validation guide by large organisations in Europe.

Good Clinical Practice (GCP)

Clinical research has a heavy requirement for computerised systems, and, in response, the European Union promulgated regulations in July 1991 to ensure that xx   **The Survive and Thrive Guide to Computer Validation**

these systems are under control and work correctly [9]. The guidelines have a section on data handling which refers to the requirements of GMP Annex 11 criteria as well as specific clinical requirements. In Section 3, the responsibilities of both the investigator and the sponsor are outlined. Clause 3.10 ranks as probably the worst computer validation regulation ever written, as it states "the sponsor must use validated error-free programs with adequate user documentation". Given this directive, we will be using pen and paper as no system will ever pass an inspection under this requirement as currently written.

GCP is still a Cinderella in computer validation circles as we have the regulations but nobody apparently willing to inspect the systems. This will change in the short to medium future, but will come as a surprise to many organisations. The term *validation* must also be used with care as it already has the meaning within clinical research and data management of "ensuring the veracity and accuracy of the clinical data themselves"—and not the computerised systems.

ISO Guide 25

One advantage in being a UKASE (United Kingdom Accreditation Service) Assessor is the opportunity to assess the impact of ISO Guide 25 [10] outside of the regulated industries. ISO Guide 25 outlines the general requirements for competence of testing and calibration laboratories. It is a voluntary quality code which takes the quality system from ISO 9000 and adapts it to laboratories. The UK interpretation of ISO Guide 25 in NAMAS M10 Section 6.11 equates computer systems with instrumentation and applies the same principles [11]. In addition it provides that "The Laboratory shall, wherever possible, ensure that computer software is fully documented and validated before use". This is a rather bald statement with little further elaboration.

However, there is a guidance document available from WELAC (Western European Laboratory Accreditation Co-operation): Appendix C. Use of Computers—General Guidance [12–13]. This document outlines many of the principles of the regulations described above, but it does not emphasize the development of computer systems, where many problems seen later in the life of systems can be prevented. There is one further NAMAS guidance document which outlines both configuration management and change control [14].

Postscript

Although there have been several European regulatory and voluntary initiatives towards validation of computerised systems, the responses of many organisations in regulated industries vary greatly from indifference to a pro-active stance. In my experience, the greatest European driver for computerised system validation is the Food and Drug Administration's Foreign Inspection Programme. Teri Stokes's book will become an invaluable tool for companies worldwide that require reliable processes for continuous validation of their computer systems.

References

1. *The Application of GLP Principles to Computer Systems*, Advisory Leaflet Number 1, Department of Health, London, 1989.

2. *The Application of GLP Principles to Computer Systems*, Advisory Leaflet Number 1, Department of Health, London, 1995.

3. *GLP Consensus Document on the Application of the Principles of GLP to Computerised Systems*, Environment Monograph No. 116, Organisation for Economic Co-operation and Development, Paris, 1995.

4. Directive 91/356/EEC *Principles and Guidelines of Good Manufacturing Practice (GMP) for Medicinal Products*, Brussels, 1991.

5. *Rules and Guidance for Pharmaceutical Manufacturers 1993* (Orange Guide), Medicines Control Agency, The Stationery Office, London, 1993.

6. *APV Guide for the Interpretation of GMP Annex 11*. See Appendix U of the GAMP Guide (reference 8).

7. *Rules and Guidance for Pharmaceutical Manufacturers and Distributors 1997*, Medicines Control Agency, The Stationery Office, London, 1997.

8. *Good Automated Manufacturing Practice Guidelines*, Version 2, International Society for Pharmaceutical Engineering, Tampa, Florida, 1996.

9. *Good Clinical Practices for Trials on Medicinal Products in the European Community*, 1991.

10. *General Requirements for the Competence of Calibration and Testing Laboratories*, ISO Guide 25, International Standards Organisation, Geneva, 3rd Edition, 1990 (currently under review).

11. NAMAS Accreditation Standard, *General Criteria of Competence for Calibration and Testing Laboratories*, Booklet M10, NAMAS Executive, Teddington, UK, 1994.

12. *WELAC Accreditation for Chemical Laboratories*, Eurachem Guidance Document NO. 1, WELAS Guidance Document, WDG 2, Laboratory of the Government Chemist, Teddington, UK, 1993.

xxii   The Survive and Thrive Guide to Computer Validation

13. *Accreditation for Chemical Laboratories* (the WELAC Guide in a different package), NIS 45, 2nd Edition, NAMAS Executive, Teddington, UK, 1996.

14. *A Guide to Managing the Configuration of Computer Systems (hardware, software and firmware) Used in NAMAS Accredited Laboratories*, NAMAS Executive, Teddington, UK, 1993.

R. D. McDowall, Ph.D.
Principal
McDowall Consulting
May 1998

JAPAN—Yasuo Bando

Yasuo Bando is manager of the Quality Assurance Regulatory Affairs Department at Takeda Pharmaceutical Company in Japan. He is chairperson of the GLP subcommittee of the Japan Society of Quality Assurance, which has a focus on the quality of computerized systems used in laboratory studies.

In recent times, computerization and issues raised by computer usage have dominated the development of information and communication technology. In the regulated industries, such as the pharmaceutical industry, computerization is especially important. The pharmaceutical industry, which affects the very lives of human beings, is regulated by Good Laboratory Practice (GLP), associated with drug safety studies; Good Clinical Practice (GCP), associated with drug clinical studies, and Good Manufacturing Practice, associated with manufacturing and quality control. Regulation of these practices is intended to assure the quality of all studies and drug products.

Because computerized systems have become heavily intertwined with good practices, it is difficult to achieve the objectives of good practices without reliable computerized systems. Thus, computerized systems that always function according to the established specifications are required. Computer validation provides a method for assuring proper operation. In Japan, computer validation has a different history and tradition for each practice.

The GLP guideline was issued in March 1982 and effective in April 1983. In May 1989, the GLP inspection of computer systems was issued as part of the GLP checklist for inspection of study facilities by a regulatory agency. In the GLP inspection of computer systems, the requirements are specified for validation of the development of computerized systems and their operation, inspections of computerized systems by a quality assurance unit, and raw data in computers; inspections by the regulatory agency are executed accordingly. The GLP inspection of computer systems does not, however, include detailed descriptions for execution of validation, and validation of computerized systems has been accepted regardless of the actual process used in executing the validation. The Japan Society of Quality Assurance, comprising industry quality assurance units, compiled a standard validation execution manual in 1994 based on *Computerized Data Systems for Nonclinical Safety Assessment—Current Concepts and Quality Assurance*, issued by the Drug Information Association in 1988. The Society has made the manual available to the public, contributed to its dissemination, and educated users.

The GCP guideline was issued in October 1989 and effective in October 1990. In March 1997, when it was revised to comply with the guidelines of the ICH (International Conference on Harmonization), validation of computerized systems for data processing became a requirement, although the MHW has not provided detailed requirements or checklists. Thus, the actual execution of computer validation has been a source of continuous controversy. In June 1997, the U.S. Food and Drug Administration (FDA) issued a draft guideline for industry computerized systems used in clinical trials, which is a useful reference on computer validation activities.

The GMP guideline for pharmaceutical products was established in August 1980 and revised in 1983; further revisions have taken place since then. The GMPs for bulk drug substances were established in July 1988. Then, in February 1992, the guideline on the control of computerized systems in drug manufacturing was established, and, in January 1993, the inspection manual for computerized systems in drug manufacturing was issued by the MHW. These two documents were intended to cope with the increasing usage of computers in process control, manufacturing administration, and quality control in drug manufacturing, since the GMP guidelines alone did not provide for appropriate development and operation of a computer system. Pharmaceutical manufacturers exporting drugs overseas also must comply with the requirements of the FDA and the EU. In Japan, the concept of validation has been well understood in GMP, and computer validation for both hardware and software has been accepted without reluctance.

In August 1997, the guideline for using electronic files for quality records of drugs and medical devices was issued. Requirements for verification, judgment, and approval of computers according to GMP were specified. Based on FDA requirements for electronic records and electronic signatures, this guideline describes the GMP requirements to which pharmaceutical facilities must adhere.

In consequence of the revised Pharmaceutical Affairs Law, which became effective in April 1997, the GLP and GCP guidelines were revised (the MHW ordinance of March 1997). In addition, reliability standards for the preparation of application dossiers were established. In auditing application dossiers, materials to prove the reliability of computer processing are required to ensure the reliability of the study. Since the reliability standards are applied to nonclinical studies, computer validation is required for all processes, from drug research and development to manufacturing.

The current understanding and implementation of computer validation differ in the areas of GLP, GCP, and GMP, and they differ among pharmaceutical firms. In general, larger, global firms have attained better understanding and implementation than smaller firms. In the future, continuous computer validation will be required in all practice areas, and the people who use, develop, and operate computerized systems in both manufacturing and quality assurance units will be expected to understand it fully.

I believe that Teri Stokes's book, covering all good practice areas and international regulations, is very timely. As chairperson of the GLP subcommittee of the Japan Society of Quality Assurance, whose purpose is to promote activities that ensure the reliability of computerized systems, I am confident that this book will become a companion for all who are involved with computerized systems in the good practice areas and contribute to the promotion of the reliability of computerized systems for achieving good practice objectives.

Yasuo Bando
Manager, Quality Assurance Regulatory Affairs Department
Takeda Pharmaceutical Company
May 1998

1. Introduction: Team and System Concepts for Computer Validation

This book is intended as a practical guide for anyone responsible for or involved in the quality assurance and validation of computerized systems. The audience is considered at two levels of the organization: the *system sponsor* and the System Validation Team or *system team* led by a *system owner*. Each chapter is structured to address the view of computer validation from both levels—the user manager's view and the perspective of the *system team* responsible for implementing and maintaining a validated system.

I. System Sponsor's Summary

What Is Computer Validation?

There have been many definitions put forward for computer validation, but from the perspective of the people who have to do the job, the following definition applies and is the one used for this book:

> **computer validation:** the practice of providing documented evidence to show that a computerized system operates *as intended* to handle and protect data or to control a work process. (T. Stokes)

Based on the good practice regulations of North America, Europe, and Japan for laboratory, clinical, and manufacturing systems used in healthcare industries, there are four major themes for computer validation. The themes or goals for computer validation are:

1

2   The Survive and Thrive Guide to Computer Validation

1. Management control of the system,

2. Integrity and security of the data handled or the process controlled,

3. Reliability of the system to perform as expected consistently, and

4. Auditable quality of the system as shown by documented evidence.

It takes a team effort to reach the goals of computer validation for strategic systems, which are often large systems supporting many user groups. The first goal, for management control, is provided by the *system sponsor*, who is a member of management designated to be the organization's senior person responsible to internal and external authorities for the system. The second and third goals are accomplished by a System Validation Team lead by a *system owner* who has been appointed by the *system sponsor*. The fourth goal is the output of the efforts to meet the first three goals, and can be assessed by a quality assurance audit or a regulatory inspection.

The System Sponsor

The *system sponsor* is the functional manager whose work team uses the computerized system for data acquisition, data handling, or process control. The *system sponsor* has company and regulatory responsibility for the data on the system or the process controlled by the system. The *system sponsor* usually carries a budgetary role for funding the system use in his or her functional area.

The primary interest of *system sponsors* is the integrity of the data on the system or the reliability of the control function the computerized system performs. They do not know or care about the technical issues of how a system works. They just want the system to do its intended job in their work process accurately, reliably, and at a reasonable cost. *System sponsors* usually pay for the purchase of special software applications required by their work process and may fund independently or collectively the purchase and ongoing support of platform systems (required computer hardware, database, network, and other components) configured to support their software applications.

System sponsors invest enormous amounts of money in computer systems every year. As the expenditures continue to grow, management in all organizations asks the question, "What is the return on this investment in computers?" In the first section of each chapter in this book, this question of return on investment (ROI) is answered with a summary discussion explaining to *system sponsors* why the chapter topic is necessary, useful, and beneficial to the organization; and thus, it is worth an investment of money, time, and other resources.

II. System Owner and System Team Discussion

The System Owner

The second major discussion section of each chapter is directed to the System Validation Team or *system team*, which is led by the *system owner*. The *system owner* is an individual designated by the *system sponsor* to be responsible for the day-to-day availability and operation of the computerized system in the work process. The *system owner* is an expert in the work process using the computer, is often not an information technology (IT) professional, and relies on a team of people with complementary skills to establish and keep the system performing as intended over time. Often the *system owner* engages the company's IT department to help in purchasing the application software and then installing, maintaining, and servicing it on a suitable platform system configured with required hardware, software, database, and network components. The *system owner* then includes the *platform supplier* as a key member of the *system team*.

The System Validation Team or System Team

The System Validation Team is assembled and led by the *system owner* on behalf of the *system sponsor*. The *system sponsor* approves and resources the *system team's* validation activities. The *system owner* selects individuals from various areas of expertise to work on a team that varies in size depending on the size and scope of the system being implemented. For a large, strategic system, the *system team* is usually composed of the following members (Figure 1.1):

- *System owner:* appointed by and reports to *system sponsor* for system purposes
- *User representative(s):* per major work group using the strategic application
- *Platform supplier(s):* IT department representative(s) providing platform systems
- *Other supplier(s):* internal or external software or service representative(s) as needed
- *Quality control (QC):* a quality professional who is separate from any quality assurance (QA) auditor for the system

Figure 1.1. System validation: people and process

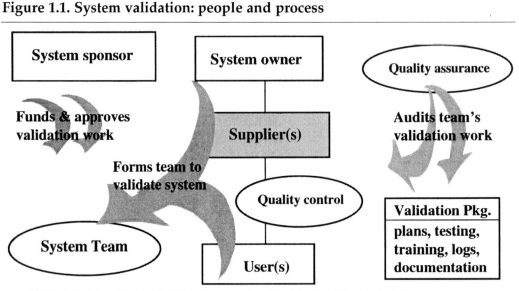

System Concepts

In order to understand the chapter discussions, it is important to define some computer system concepts that are common to all topics in this book. These concepts are based upon and adapted from those published by the Computer Systems Validation Committee (CSVC) of the U.S. Pharmaceutical Manufacturers Association (PMA) in the 1980s.[1]

As shown in Figure 1.2, the CSVC used a manufacturing example and identified a **computer system** composed of hardware and software that worked along with a **process system** composed of people, procedures, and equipment to

Figure 1.2. Computer system environment

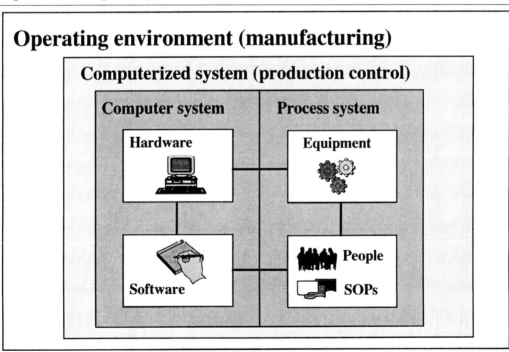

[1]. PMA/CSVC. Validation Concepts for Computer Systems Used in the Manufacture of Drug Products, *Pharm. Technol.* 10 (5):24–34, 1986.

perform a business function. The computer system and the process system worked together to form a **computerized system**, such as a production control system. The **computerized system** then worked within an **operating environment** or business area of the company, such as product manufacturing.

Figure 1.2 is important to validation work because the goal of computer validation is to show that a *computerized system* performs as intended in its *operating environment*. The System Validation Team includes *user representatives* who understand the demands of the operating environment and can help test the system to be sure it meets the demands of its real-world situation. As later chapters will explain, this is different from the verification work performed by a software design team who tests the application to see if it meets the criteria specified in its design description.

A further adaptation of the PMA model is needed to help non-IT professionals on the System Team understand how hardware and software are configured and where to focus their validation efforts. As shown in Figure 1.3, the software application system is the software code that interacts with people, processes, and equipment to perform real work in the business process. This is the *user's* view of the computerized system; it is also the *system sponsor's* major interest, because work performed by the software application in the operating environment is the business reason for investing in the system in the first place.

There are many ways a software application can function in a business process. It may collect data from on-line instruments or keyboard input by people; it may control a process by turning valves on or off; or it may release material from inventory quarantine to be used in production. It may perform various calculations and graphing procedures to support human decisions, or it may send data and messages to other locations or parts of the process to authorize continued actions by people or equipment. In short, the software application is the part of a computerized system whose intended purpose can have a direct impact on the safety, efficacy, and quality of the product or process being supported by the computerized system, or it may have

Figure 1.3. Software application system

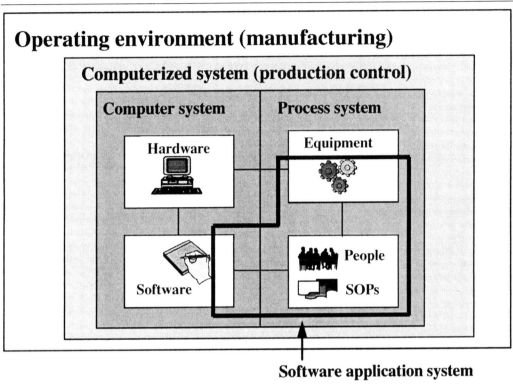

a direct impact on the safety of the *user* working in the operating environment.

Every software application has a specific set of functions that are unique to its intended purpose; however, no application is able to operate totally on its own. It needs a specific set or "configuration" of computer hardware, operating system, software tools, database engine, storage disks, network infrastructure, and other components to allow it to function as intended. This configuration of required components is called a *platform system* and is usually supplied by the company's IT department as a service to the functional business units (Figure 1.4).

The software application resides on a *platform system*. It can be located in the immediate area of the operating

Figure 1.4. The platform system

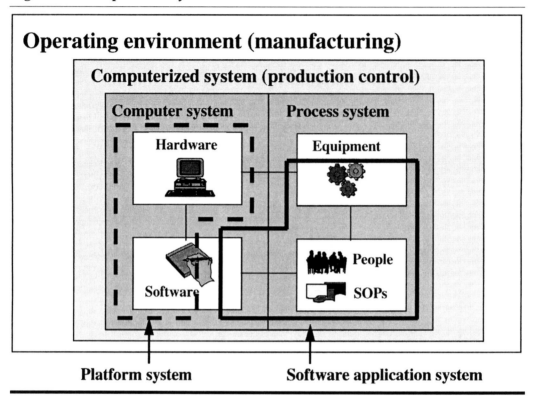

environment or in the company's data center with the application being called and used over a network. Sometimes, the host *platform system* is even in another country, and the application is called by personal computer (PC) over a wide area network (WAN) to allow people to input data and print reports locally.

To scope *system team* efforts, it is important to identify and separate the software application from the *platform system*. Then a reasonable strategy for validation actions can be developed for each. If a platform system is used by several strategic applications, then one separate validation testing of the platform system should suffice for all applications using it. During the validation testing of each application, further testing of the platform system will occur by default

Team and System Concepts for Computer Validation

and should identify any special needs on a per-application basis that might have been missed in the general platform system testing.

Quality Concepts for Computerized Systems

Throughout this book and across many regulations and guidelines, the concepts for quality in computerized systems have several core themes. These themes are listed in Figure 1.5 and actually make up a good list of titles for system standard operating procedure (SOP) topics. The associated picture shows the major components of a strategic manufacturing system known as a supervisory control and data acquisition (SCADA) system that would require validation.

Figure 1.5. Computer system quality concepts

Quality Assurance
- Training/SOPs
- Change control
- Backup/recovery
- System testing
- Service/support
- Logs & records
- Problem/help
- System/data security

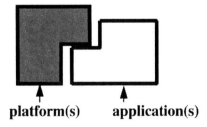

In Figure 1.5, the SCADA host application sits on a central platform system and accepts input from multiple programmable logic controllers (PLCs). The PLCs are hardware devices that use ladder logic as their software application to gather information from instruments and machines on a production line. The PLCs gather data such as temperature and pressure readings and send them to the SCADA host application. The SCADA host application then stores, calculates, and graphs the input to help production workers control the production process. Often, the SCADA host will send commands by itself to other PLCs to open and close valves or take other action based on the input it receives and the rules programmed into its host software. Validating a SCADA system requires that testing, calibration, and quality activities be performed on both the SCADA host and its associated PLCs. All four components shown need to work properly for the production process to stay in control.

To assure the quality of any computerized system, it is important to have proper training materials and a training plan for new system users and support personnel. Both groups also need to have SOPs written and available in their working area to provide clear instructions for human interaction with the system. Such guidance helps to prevent system failure due to human error.

Any change to the platform components or software application must take place in a controlled manner. This means that any request for change should be in writing, and the actions taken should also be in writing and recorded in a system logbook. Any changes to solve a problem with the system or to add new functions to the system should be documented in the system's Change Log.

A procedure should exist and be exercised for regular backup of the system and its data and for recovery from unexpected shutdown and disaster situations. System testing should be planned and documented with written scripts and the results recorded in logs. Records of ongoing service and support of the platform components and application software should be kept. Such logs and records need to be kept up-to-date and need to be made available for audit purposes.

System *users* should have a documented process for obtaining help in operating the system and for where to bring problems for resolution. They should also be taught the policy and procedures for system and data security. Some key concepts for data and system security are shown in Figure 1.6.

There should be an SOP written to inform users and support personnel about the actions to be taken to ensure the physical, logical, and network security of the computerized systems and data with which they work. The physical aspects of system and data security can be addressed with instructions for care in the handling of diskettes and tapes; locked doors, drawers, and cabinets; restricted access to

Figure 1.6. Data and system security concepts

Security
- SOP
- Physical
- Logical
- Network

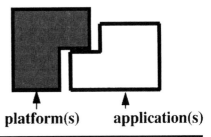

12 The Survive and Thrive Guide to Computer Validation

computer areas; and restricted use of network modems for the Internet.

The careful use, protection, and changing of passwords and personal codes, together with the use of tools such as virus checkers, can help with the logical security of the system and its data. The basic message is that security is everyone's job. Data center personnel are usually trained in such matters and follow security practices as normal work practice. Application users operating personal computers (PCs) in more open environments are often not aware of security requirements. They need a written SOP and security training to help guide them in this matter.

III. Conclusion

Why Validate?

With these basic concepts in mind, *sponsors, owners,* and *system teams* should be able to proceed through the rest of this book, reading the chapters in any sequence relevant to their current interest. Each chapter is self-contained for its validation topic. Experience has shown certain regulatory documents to be particularly useful to system teams. These documents from various international authorities have been included in Chapters 13–15 for convenient reference to the original text.

The one question that perhaps needs to be raised in conclusion is, "Why should computer validation be performed at all?" It takes time, planning, and people, and it costs money across the whole lifetime of a computerized system. What is the ROI on this cost of validation? The reason and return are summed up when a *system sponsor* and *system owner* are able to respond to internal auditors or regulatory inspectors and say "Yes" to all six questions listed in Figure 1.7 with evidence to support their positive answers.

Figure 1.7. Why perform computer validation?

- Can you trust your electronic data?
- Can you measure the quality return on your IT investment?
- Are you in control of your automated processes?
- Can you recover from a physical or electronic disaster?
- Is your important data protected?
- Can your systems pass regulatory inspection?

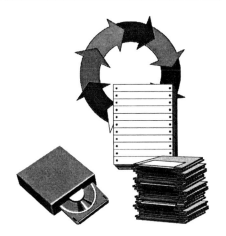

2. Managing System Life Cycles

I. System Sponsor's Summary

Return on Investment

A *system sponsor* carries both company and regulatory responsibility for the data on a computerized system and the system's ability to control a process or handle data as intended. The *system sponsor* is responsible for a firm's ROI from the computerized system. The *sponsor's* goal is to have the system perform its intended job in the work process accurately, reliably, and at a reasonable cost. In order to achieve a good ROI, it is necessary to manage a strategic computerized system with the same care as with any other priority project. This is accomplished by appointing a *system owner* as project manager for the whole life cycle of the computerized system.

System Life Cycle and Owner Selection

Figure 2.1 shows the typical life cycle for a computerized system. It begins with the first idea for a system (Phase 1)—performing a Needs Analysis and writing a proposal to purchase the system. In Phase 2, the proposal is refined into a *user requirements specification* (URS), which is then used as input for the *system development life cycle* (SDLC) in Phases 3–5. After being designed, built, and tested by the *supplier*, the system is released to the *owner's* site for commissioning, operation, and maintenance. Eventually, the system moves on to Phase 9 for retirement and replacement. It is important that *system sponsors* recognize the total *system life cycle*

Figure 2.1. System life cycle: phases/activities

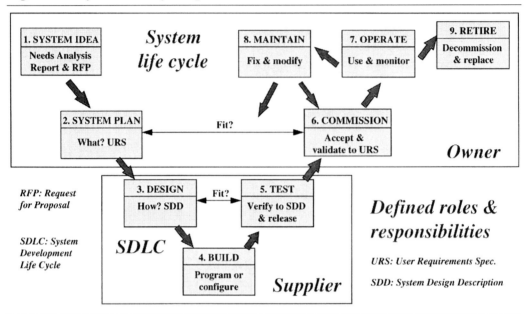

(Phases 1–9) as a multiyear information technology (IT) project and that they choose a *system owner* who can apply project management skills to the role and can give proactive leadership to the *system team*.

When selecting a *system owner*, the *sponsor* should look for good project management and leadership skills and a thorough understanding of the work process using the computerized system. Extensive IT experience is not a critical factor and can be supplied by other team members. The selected *owner* can contract with internal or external IT professionals to provide platform systems and other IT services, as well as fill any technical requirements for the *system team*.

II. System Owner and System Team Discussion

Computer validation is a journey, not a destination. In fact, it is a journey that can have many repeating loops in its path. The full *system life cycle* is shown as a straightforward march from Phase 1 through to Phase 9 in Figure 2.1. For some custom-built software applications, however, the SDLC can be executed with many iterations of Steps 2–6 to pilot software approaches before a final system is accepted and used in operation.

During operation and maintenance of a system (Phases 7 and 8), problem resolutions and minor fixes may cycle back to retesting in Phase 6, or major modifications may cycle back to the supplier starting at a modified Phase 2–3. When the system is retired, a whole new life cycle begins following a decommission of the old system and the execution of a transition plan to migrate data and operations to the new replacement system.

It is the responsibility of the *system owner* and *system team* to define and develop the procedures and documented evidence necessary to keep the system under control and to protect the integrity of any data it handles throughout its life cycle. In an ideal world, the *system owner* is appointed and forms a *system team* as part of Phase 1 when the Needs Analysis is being performed. The *system team* can then input requirements for quality control and validation into the Needs Analysis, the request for proposal (RFP), and the URS to ensure that they are built into the system from the very start and will not have to be retrofitted into the system at Phase 6.

Phase 1. System Idea

Needs Analysis Report

The life of a system begins with an effort to understand the needs of the business process for data handling, information processing, and/or automated controls. A good way to gain such understanding is through performing a Needs Analysis. In this analysis, people close to the work activity are interviewed about the flow of information through the business process and the current types and sources of critical data. From interview results, several different maps can be plotted to show where critical data are generated (by which person or device), where it goes to next, how it is transformed (calculated, graphed, edited), who approves it, who stores it, who has access to it, and how the information is retrieved and sent to the next part of the business process.

When conducting such interviews, it is important to go beyond department heads and include daily and alternate shift workers in the Needs Analysis discussions. It is not uncommon for managers to give one "official" view of information flow and discover later that the real work is performed along quite a different path by the people who have to make things happen in the actual business process.

In working with the Needs Analysis Report, the *system team* should look for ways to improve the current process when moving to a computerized system. After plotting the current data handling situation, the team should consider how computerization could improve the work process with new ways to process information in parallel; to merge phone, fax, paper, and electronic input; and to create more efficient communication paths to help reduce business cycle times. Increased productivity is the goal for introducing a new system, not faster implementation of current inefficiencies.

Among the needs to be analyzed and included in the report are the system quality assurance and security concepts discussed in Chapter 1. Program checks for critical data and security protection, with password and code control for electronic signatures, can ensure data integrity and system security for critical information. Identifying such needs at the start can save a lot of time and money over trying to add them in later.

Due consideration should also be given to any external standards or regulatory requirements required by the work process, such as ISO 9000 (International Organization for Standardization) or Good Manufacturing Practice (GMP), Good Laboratory Practice (GLP), and Good Clinical Practice (GCP), required by regulators of the healthcare industries. A generic term to use for all the good practices is GXP, where X stands for M, L, C, or any other regulated requirement.

Managing System Life Cycles   19

Request for Proposal (RFP)

The second step in defining the system idea is to take the business needs from the analysis report and translate them into system requirements that potential suppliers can understand. A good RFP begins with a concise description of the business process to be computerized and a definition of the business objectives for the prospective system. These include the metrics against which the *sponsor* will be measured for the company's investment in purchasing the new system. Such metrics could be the elimination of rework due to lost requisition slips or the reduction of cycle time within the department.

The RFP then describes the business needs in terms of critical data handling requirements, such as the following:

- Maps of critical data flow through the business process and of work functions to be handled by the new system

- Data types (text, voice, graphics, video, image) and amount (per day, week, month)

- Sources of data (keyboard, modem, instrument, device, voice, keypad, or fax)

- Data transformation needs (calculations, graphing, statistical analysis)

- Number and type of users (concurrent, special, high or low volume)

- Database needs (relational, structured, object oriented); existing database(s) to be used

- Compatibility needs (existing systems to be connected, type of connection, type of communication required, such as text, image, signal)

- Network needs (internal or external to the department, internal or external to the site)

- Security needs (password, key code, audit trail, automated backup, virus checking)

- Validation needs (audit of supplier's QA activities during SDLC, verification testing, specific GXP regulation(s) to be applied)

20   The Survive and Thrive Guide to Computer Validation

- Support, maintenance, and training needs (help desk, on-site repair coverage, courses)

It then continues with whatever business terms and conditions normally apply to the company's purchasing practices. An excellent guide for writing software development contracts and for defining quality needs with software suppliers is found in the ISO 9000-3 standard. Section 5.2.2 of ISO 9000-3 discusses important contract items related to quality, which are quoted in Figure 2.2.[1]

Phase 2. System Plan

Choosing the supplier for a strategic system is an important decision and has a long-term impact on the life cycle activities of the *system owner* and *system team*. The Institute of Electrical and Electronic Engineers, Inc. (IEEE) has published a guidance document with a nine-step model for the acquisition of software (IEEE Standard 1062-1993). Table 2.1 gives an overview of the nine steps in the life cycle of purchasing a system and shows related GXP validation activities to be performed at each step.[2]

User Requirements Specification (URS)

Once a supplier has been chosen, the Needs Analysis Report, RFP, and Supplier's Proposal can be molded into a URS that more exactly describes *what* the new system is expected to do in its operating environment. Each functional requirement must be written in such a way that it is measurable by some means of testing, because the URS now becomes the benchmark for acceptance and validation testing performed during commissioning in Phase 6 of the *system life cycle*.

---

1. International Standard ISO 9000-3, Quality Management and Quality Assurance Standards—Part 3: Guidelines for the Application of ISO 9001 to the Development, Supply, and Maintenance of Software, 1st ed. (International Organization for Standardization, Geneva), p. 4 (1991-06-01).

2. IEEE Recommended Practice for Software Acquisition: Std. 1062-1993 (The Institute for Electrical and Electronic Engineers, Inc., Piscataway, NJ: 1993), p. 6.

Managing System Life Cycles **21**

Figure 2.2. Contract items on quality: ISO 9000-3, Sections 5.2.2 and 5.9.1

5.2.2 Contract items on quality

Among others, the following items are frequently found to be relevant in the contract:

a)   acceptance criteria;

b)   handling of the changes in purchaser's requirements during the development;

c)   handling of problems detected after acceptance, including quality-related claims and purchaser complaints;

d)   activities carried out by the purchaser, especially the purchaser's role in requirements specification, installation and acceptance;

e)   facilities, tools and software items to be provided by the purchaser;

f)   standards and procedures to be used;

g)   replication requirements (see 5.9).

5.9.1 Replication

Replication is a step which should be conducted prior to delivery. In providing for replication, consideration should be given to the following:

a)   the number of copies of each software item to be delivered

b)   the type of media for each software item, including format and version, in human-readable form;

c)   the stipulation of required documentation such as manuals and user guides;

d)   copyright and licensing concerns addressed and agreed to;

e)   custody of master and back-up copies where applicable, including disaster recovery plans;

f)   the period of obligation of the supplier to supply copies.

Extra time spent to develop a strong URS will be repaid many times over with a smoother development cycle, better product fit to the business process, and clearer testing strategies for acceptance and validation in the Phase 6 commissioning process. A common system RFP requirement is that it be "user-friendly," but such words do not describe URS-measurable attributes for what "user-friendly" means. The URS should define "user-friendly" with such

22 The Survive and Thrive Guide to Computer Validation

Table 2.1. IEEE Software Acquisition Model (Std. 1062-1993) and Related GXP Activities

Life Cycle of a System Purchase	Nine Steps in the Acquisition Process		Related GXP Validation Activities	
I. Planning	1.	Planning organizational strategy	1.	Analyze user needs and determine GXP status of data to be handled by software.
	2.	Implementing organization's process	2.	Apply computer validation SOPs and GXP quality regulations to company's purchasing process.
	3.	Determining software requirements	3.	Develop RFP to include a written description of software functions, GXP quality needs, acceptance criteria, and validation process.
II. Contracting	4.	Identifying potential suppliers	4.	Select candidates who will: demonstrate their software, provide documentation for their software, and provide formal proposals.
	5.	Preparing contract requirements	5.	Develop Service Level Agreement (SLA) contract to include QA audits, documented software testing, payments tied to performance milestones, and software documentation sets.
	6.	Evaluating proposals and selecting the supplier	6.	Select a qualified supplier with a documented software QA process and negotiate SLA contract. Review contract with legal counsel.

Continued on next page.

Continued from previous page.

Life Cycle of a System Purchase	Nine Steps in the Acquisition Process		Related GXP Validation Activities	
III. Product Implementation	7.	Managing supplier performance	7.	Monitor supplier's performance to all milestones and approv e work segments. Provide all of the purchaser's deliverables to the supplier when needed.
IV. Product Acceptance	8.	Accept the product	8.	Review and test product to written Validation Plan and Test Plan procedures to certify that all discrepancies are corrected and all acceptance criteria are satisfied.
V. Follow-on	9.	Using the software	9.	Establish change control and maintenance logs, ongoing user training and periodic re-testing as per Validation Plan.

specifications as "new system users must be trainable in two to four hours" or "system must be available through company's current graphical user interface (GUI)" or "system must accept certain local language character sets."

For off-the-shelf (OTS) components of a system, such as Microsoft Office for Windows '95, the SDLC remains invisible to the *system owner* and *system team*. For custom-built or highly modified components and software application systems, the URS provides a fixed user description as input to the SDLC design phase.

Phase 3. Design

System Design Description (SDD)

The supplier uses a URS as a functional model for writing a technical system design description (SDD). The SDD document defines the structural blueprint for *how* to build a system to perform the functions described in the URS. It becomes the common standard for the supplier's software engineering team to use in their work of building and testing the system. Concerns about the technical feasibility of certain URS items or frequent changes to the URS content by an undecided *owner* need to be discussed and cleared in this phase, not left to later phases.

Just as in house construction, it is very costly to try to build a software application system with a changing set of "blueprints." Having to rip out, rework, and retrofit various units of system code can cause chaos in the code structure, resulting in broken module interfaces; blind alleys in data paths; and unexpected, intermittent disruption in performance of various subunits. The same problems can arise if there is no written SDD and a group of programmers write individual pieces of the system without a coherent architecture established in the beginning for the whole design.

When an *owner* is trying to use new technology or computerize a new process, there may be a need to take an experimental approach to developing the system, and a spiral or iterative design process is used. In this case, the *owner* and the supplier are working together to do something new and innovative, and there may be several cycles of URS and SDD development, resulting in several pilot systems being built and tested before the final system is achieved. Good practice in software and system engineering requires a documented process for every step of development (Phases 3–5) and every version of product developed (Figure 2.3).

The use of multicycle design methods still requires documented version control and should never be allowed as an excuse for poor software engineering documentation practices. Executing multiple build cycles without proper

Figure 2.3. System development life cycle (SDLC)

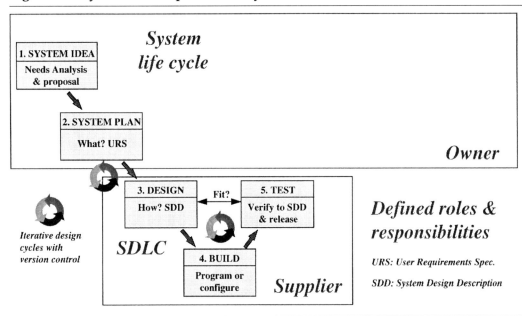

documentation can result in software code that is incapable of being fully documented or properly serviced; thus, it is not validatable and usable for strategic systems or regulated environments.

Phase 4. Build

Program New Code or Configure Adjustable Code

When Phases 1–3 have been thoughtfully and carefully executed, the programming or configuring of system code is very straightforward and takes far less time than expected. If users keep changing their functional demands in the URS or a supplier writes an incomplete SDD, rework of the code can become endless, and many problems or bugs can be introduced into the system. Establishing a standard set of naming conventions, coding standards, and documentation requirements per project keeps all programmers working in a consistent way and improves the reliability and performance of a system.

26 The Survive and Thrive Guide to Computer Validation

Adhering to such documented programming standards will make Phase 8 maintenance and support work less complicated. New code will fit better with the original code and be less likely to introduce more problems than it solves when programmers adding fixes or modifications to a system can use the same standards as the original. **Note:** It is normal for programmers to complain about documenting their code until they are the ones who have to go back and troubleshoot or modify it. Then they are very happy that they left notes about how the code was structured.

Phase 5. Test

Verification to SDD and Release to Owner

For a large, software development project, there are many levels of testing performed during the SDLC. The first level of testing is performed by programmers doing their own testing as they write the code and then try it to see if it works properly. As some small unit of code has been written, the second level of SDLC testing occurs when the original programmer gives the new code to a colleague to test it and check to see if it works properly. This colleague testing is sometimes called "peer review," and it can have different degrees of formality.

As major units of the system functions are completed, they are tested more formally on a unit-by-unit basis called "unit testing." One formal method for doing such testing is to conduct a code "walk-through." In this process, the programmer presents his or her code to a group of design team members who review the code line by line and give comment and feedback. Finally, all the units are put together, and the system is tested as an whole system. This last level of testing is called "integrated testing." Its goal is to be sure that all of the interactions and interdependencies between and among the various parts of the system operate as intended in the SDD.

Testing performed during the SDLC is focused on the structural integrity of the software. This means that the software code is tested for compliance to its design description (SDD) and answers the question "**Has the software been built right?**" Did the programmers follow the blueprints and build what the supplier was contracted to build? Much of this testing is "white box" testing, which means that the system is being tested for its functions based on known structural pathways in the code.

Understanding the system fit to the SDD is the goal of SDLC testing and is part of the supplier's verification process prior to releasing the system for shipment to its new *owner*. When the SDD is an accurate technical representation of the functions specified by the URS, and the URS truly reflects the needs of the business process, the new system released to the *owner* should work well upon installation in its operating environment.

Phase 6. Commission

System Acceptance

The commissioning process involves two levels of testing a new system and answers the question "**Has the right software been built?**" The first level of system checking is acceptance testing. The major criteria for acceptance testing should be stated in the supplier's contract. Once the system has been set up at the *owner's* site, the *system team* executes and documents Installation Qualification (IQ) and Operational Qualification (OQ) testing.

During IQ testing, the physical and logical configuration of the system is checked for compliance to the supplier's technical specifications for the application and its platform components. Specific requirements for power supply, memory capacity, versions of platform software, network protocols, and other specifications (such as temperature, humidity, and dust control) must be checked and recorded as met.

During OQ testing, the *owner* can assume (based on vendor audits) that extensive SDLC testing of the system structure has been performed. The *owner* checks to be sure that all of the user functions required by the URS are present and operational. The system is then tested for its ability to function properly within the normal operational limits set by the URS for major units of the application (Figure 2.4).

Validation to URS and Release for Active Use

For strategic systems and those systems expected to operate in regulated areas, further testing must be performed and controls established prior to releasing the system for active use. A Validation Plan is written that requires IQ, OQ, and Performance Qualification (PQ) testing be performed according to a written test plan, using written test scripts with logs for recording test results. System functions are challenged to see if they operate as intended under normal, problem, and stress situations in the work process.

The goal of validation testing by the *owner* and *system team* is to check the operational fit of the delivered system to the URS requirements, the system documentation descriptions

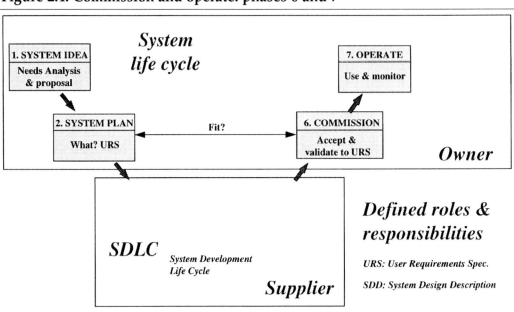

Figure 2.4. Commission and operate: phases 6 and 7

in user materials, regulatory requirements, any other standards for the business process, and the usual range of problems and misadventures encountered in the real-world operating environment. This type of testing is called "black box" testing, where specific inputs to the system are expected to produce known outputs. Normal data should produce routine functional output, and problem data should be handled with appropriate error messages and screens. Stress conditions should trigger appropriate alarms. It is the function or action of the system and not the structure of the code that is the focus of "black box" testing. It answers the question, **"Does the system perform as expected in a given situation?"**

A Test Summary Report is then developed to evaluate all testing activities and to provide a statement of the system's fitness for use in the regulated business process. When training materials, user SOPs, system SOPs, and other elements of a system validation package have been assembled, a Validation Summary Report is written, and a statement releasing the system for validated use in the business process is signed by the *system owner* and *sponsor*. The system then moves into its operation phase.

Phase 7. Operate

Use and Monitor

Operating a validated system requires a disciplined approach, which means a documented approach, to the tasks of operating the system according to system SOPs and monitoring its performance over time by maintaining log records for the following:

- Problem resolution

- Calibration and QC activities on the system

- Training new users prior to system use

- Control of any changes to the system

- Security, backup, and recovery of the application and platform systems

The Survive and Thrive Guide to Computer Validation

- Control of access and edits to critical data handled by the system

Keeping a system in a validated state is an ongoing process of QA activities that must be integrated into the normal workflow of using the system. System and user SOPs provide the mechanism for standardizing the human interaction with the system in order to maintain its validation status during ongoing operation. The use of standard forms, reports, and logbooks can make system monitoring and quality practices automatic for system users and support personnel. Such practices provide documented evidence suitable for audit and inspection purposes.

Phase 8. Maintain

Fix and Modify

Maintaining a validated system requires documenting normal service and support activities and providing for version control of updates to system documentation and validation package documents when changes are made to fix or modify the software application or key components of the platform system supporting it. The original test plan for the system should define what constitutes a major, moderate, or minor change to the system and should specify the corresponding amount of retesting to be performed based on the degree of change. Minor fixes can be made in the *owner's* organization, but "fatal" errors or major system crashes may have to be referred back to the supplier's organization for resolution and require some new commissioning activity before returning on-line (Figure 2.5).

It is normal for any large, complex software application to experience some problems when it encounters unexpected stresses in the *owner's* real working environment; then the need arises to fix or modify system code. The larger the number of customers there are for a particular system, the more likely it is that other previous *owners* have discovered the worst bugs. The supplier may have already fixed them or developed and installed alternate solutions to the latest version just purchased.

Figure 2.5. Operate and maintain: phases 7 and 8

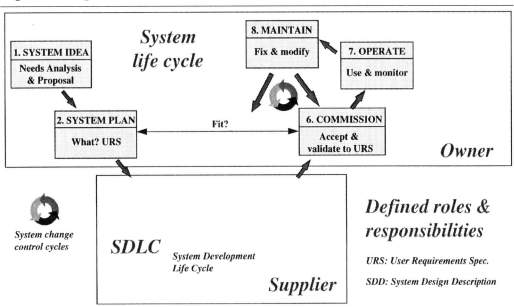

For custom-built, single-owner systems, the opportunity for problem-solving after the start of operational use is much higher. The number and severity of problems encountered and the time required to resolve them is in inverse proportion to the time and care taken to develop the URS and SDD for the system. Making adjustments at the original URS/SDD level is less costly by orders of magnitude than making modifications to fix functions after the system is operational. Later stage modifications may interrupt the business process itself during system downtime, causing even more expense.

Phase 9. Retire

Decommission and Replace

The retirement and replacement of a validated system may be initiated for any of the following reasons:

- The supplier releases a major new version of the current system.

- The supplier discontinues support for the installed version of the current system.

- There is a change of operating system and/or database versions in the platform system that is incompatible with the current system.

- A different system is required to handle a revamped work process requiring new functions to be computerized.

- The current system has insufficient capacity for the *user's* needs.

At some point, the cost to maintain a mature system becomes more than the cost to replace it. Commercial software suppliers continue to update their products and eventually stop supporting older versions. Other times, the *owner's* business process changes to such an extent and modification costs become so high that a new system is recommended.

It is important to remember that a validated system operating in a regulated environment can never be allowed to just "die." It is "retired" by being decommissioned into an archived status. A transition plan is developed to migrate its functions and critical data into the early planning phases of the new system's life cycle (Figure 2.6).

A critical component of any Needs Analysis for a new system is the identification of current systems whose functions and data need to make the transition into the new system's operation. Preparing a written Transition Plan for each retiring or legacy system as part of the planning phase for the new system helps the *owner* and *system team* prepare the *users* for changes to come and better identifies the resources required to commission the new system and retire the legacy ones.

Since validated systems operate in strategic functions and handle critical data, documented attention must be paid to continuity of the business process and integrity of

Figure 2.6. System retirement and replacement

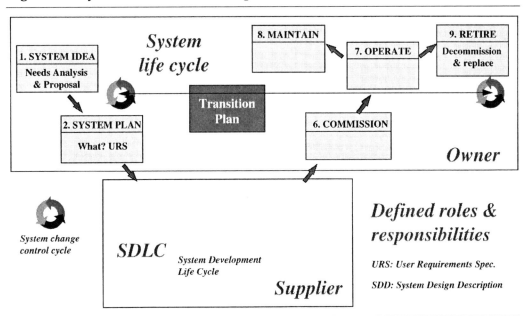

regulated data during transition activities. Such documented attention is defined in a written Transition Plan that should address the following items:

- Configuration of application and platform systems to be retired (legacy system)
- Description of critical data files to be moved into archive status (legacy data)
- Description of archival process for legacy systems and legacy data
- Description of critical data files to be moved into the new system environment (active data)
- Plan for pre- and postmove testing of active data as it migrates to the new system environment
- Plan for pre- and postmove testing of data handling interfaces and interactions with other systems in the business process

34   The Survive and Thrive Guide to Computer Validation

A final Transition Summary Report is written by the *system team* to review the results of all Transition Plan activities. This report includes a statement about the validated archival status for the legacy system and legacy data and a *system owner's* release of active data to the new system in a validated state. One copy of the Transition Summary Report is archived with the Transition Plan in the Validation Package of the legacy system. A second copy of the report becomes part of the Validation Package for the new system.

III. Conclusion

Validation Is a Lifetime Process for a Regulated System

The *owner* of a validated system is responsible for the whole life cycle of that system, from the first planning stages to its retirement, archival, and replacement with a new system. When commercial software applications are purchased and used without extensive modification, the SDLC activities are not seen or controlled by the *system owner*. With such off-the-shelf systems, the *owner* and *system team* keep a focus on non-SDLC phases of the system life cycle.

Custom-Built Systems Increase the Owner's Life Cycle Work

When the software application system is custom-built or requires major reconfiguration and modification, the *owner* must audit and monitor the supplier's quality practices during the SDLC as well as keep a focus on the rest of the system life cycle phases. When a *system owner* decides to write his or her own software application, then full responsibility for the SDLC is included in the *owner's* and *system team's* work for computer validation (Figure 2.7).

Managing System Life Cycles   35

Figure 2.7. External and internal system development

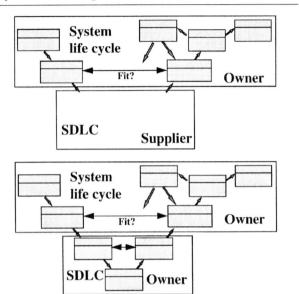

System owner's validation focus when system comes from external suppliers—only audit SDLC.

System life cycles

System owner's validation focus when system comes from internal suppliers—full responsibility for SDLC.

3. The Supplier's Verification Package

I. System Sponsor's Summary

The supplier of a regulated software application or custom-built computerized system is responsible for providing documented evidence of the QA and QC activities performed during the system development life cycle (SDLC). The supplier also provides support for installation, training, and maintenance of the system during other life cycle phases (Figure 3.1). Commercial suppliers to pharmaceutical and other regulated industries are expected to be ready to host audits of their quality practices as part of a vendor qualification process and later as part of the project and system management practices. *Sponsors* should ensure that vendor support for SDLC audit and regulatory inspection is included in contract terms.

Internal or external suppliers of custom-built or highly modified software for regulated applications must be prepared to work within a documented QA framework. One of the best ways to accomplish this is for the supplier to define, develop, and maintain a supplier's *verification package* of documented evidence that establishes the quality of the SDLC and its product. The standard content for such a *verification package* is shown in Figure 3.2. These are items that the *sponsor's* QA organization should be able to examine during any audit of the supplier. Sometimes, *sponsors* will find that external suppliers are better prepared than internal suppliers to provide such package items; this often leads to a "buy" rather than "make" decision for strategic systems.

Figure 3.1. System supplier's verification focus

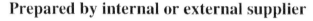

Figure 3.2. Supplier's verification package

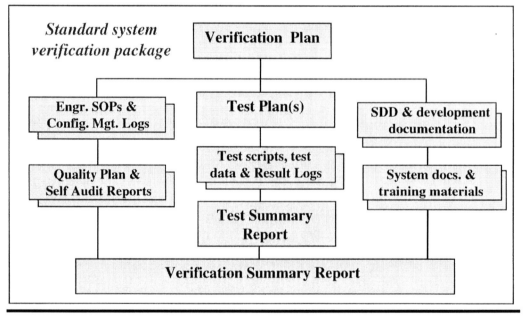

The Supplier's Verification Package **39**

Suppliers of off-the-shelf (OTS) software applications and computerized systems used across many industries such as Microsoft Office in Windows '95 usually are not aware of and do not plan for audit and inspection needs. Their products are used by so many thousands of users that any fatal flaws are quickly found and resolved with fixes.

When using such OTS systems in regulated activities, it is important to separate the general product code from any element which has been modified or configured to perform a specific GXP task. Using a spreadsheet example, it is not the Excel application or Windows '95 that is to be verified. It is rather the individual spreadsheet, designed for a regulated purpose, and written using Excel, that needs to be tested to document its quality for audit and inspection purposes.

II. System Owner and System Team Discussion

The internal or external supplier of a regulated software application or computerized system must have a documented quality process for the SDLC in order for a *system owner* and *system team* to be able to validate the installed final product. Standard items to be included in a documented quality process are shown in Figure 3.2. The supplier's responsibility to provide documented verification is also described in the International Standard ISO 9000-3 guideline, section 4.1.1.2.2 as follows:[1]

> *Verification Resources and Personnel*
> The supplier shall identify in-house verification requirements, provide adequate resources and assign trained personnel for verification activities. Verification activities shall include inspection, test and monitoring of the design, production, installation and servicing processes and/or product. Design reviews and audits of the quality system, processes

---

1. International Standard ISO 9000-3, Quality Management and Quality Assurance Standards—Part 3: Guidelines for the Application of ISO 9001 to the Development, Supply, and Maintenance of Software, 1st ed. (International Organization for Standardization, Geneva), p. 2 (1991-06-01).

and/or product shall be carried out by personnel independent of those having direct responsibility for the work being performed.

This standard requires that the supplier's management define in writing its policy and objectives for quality, its commitment to quality, and its follow-through for implementing and maintaining the policy at all levels of the organization. An important part of the follow-through is the delegation of authority, along with responsibility for personnel who manage, perform, and verify work affecting quality. This is particularly important for personnel who need the organizational freedom to do the following:[2]

a) initiate action to prevent the occurrence of product nonconformity

b) identify and record any product quality problems

c) initiate, recommend, or provide solutions through designated channels

d) verify the implementation of solutions

e) control further processing, delivery or installation of nonconforming product until the deficiency or unsatisfactory condition has been corrected.

The Purchaser's Representative

The ISO 9000-3 standard identifies the other half of the supplier's relationship to be the purchaser and assigns quality responsibilities for the purchaser as well. The *system sponsor* and *owner* are expected to cooperate with the supplier by providing all necessary information in a timely manner and resolving pending issues. A purchaser's representative is to be assigned and given the responsibility and authority for dealing with the supplier on contractual matters such as the following:[3]

---

2. Ibid.
3. Ibid.

a) defining the purchaser's requirements to the supplier

b) answering questions from the supplier

c) approving the supplier's proposals

d) concluding agreements with the supplier

e) ensuring the purchaser's organization observes the agreements made with the supplier

f) defining acceptance criteria and procedures

g) dealing with the purchaser-supplied software items that are found unsuitable for use

This representative role can be played by the *system owner* or be delegated by the *owner* to an IT professional on the *system team*. The activity of "defining the purchaser's requirements" should be one of clarifying items in the request for proposal (RFP) and/or user requirements specification (URS). The purchaser's representative also attends regular joint meetings to review the software conformance to URS requirements, the results of verification testing, and acceptance testing results. The results of such reviews should be agreed and documented and then become part of the self-audit report files for the project's *verification package* as shown in Figure 3.2.

The Supplier's Representative

An important part of the purchasing process for a strategic, custom-built system is the supplier's appointment of a "mutual success representative" as a single interface for working with the purchaser's representative. This individual should be oriented more toward project management than sales and have access to all areas of the supplier's organization and the project's technical team. This person's decision-making authority should be clearly understood and should be as comprehensive as possible so that resolving project issues is not delayed by many levels of approval.

Frequent changes in the purchaser and/or supplier representatives is a recipe for mutual disaster on a project.

42 The Survive and Thrive Guide to Computer Validation

Continuity of personnel leads to continuity in expectations and a stronger mutual understanding on both sides of the relationship so that SDLC activities proceed according to agreed standards and are documented in an auditable fashion. The documentation that relates to controlling the SDLC quality process are shown in Figure 3.3. These include the Verification Plan, engineering SOPs, configuration management logs, the system design description (SDD), development documentation, the quality plan, and Self-Audit Reports.

Supplier's Verification Plan

The quality verification framework for any system development project is defined in the Verification Plan for the system. This document describes the standard practices to be used for designing, building, and testing the system and

Figure 3.3. Supplier's SDLC quality assurance

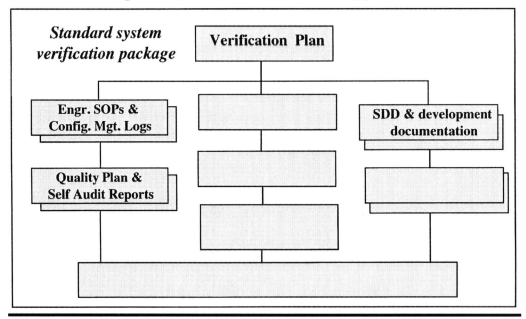

The Supplier's Verification Package   43

the content of various items required for the *verification package*. It also assigns roles and responsibilities in the supplier's organization for implementing all parts of the plan throughout the system's SDLC. In the end, the plan requires a Verification Summary Report of all quality activities carried out under the plan.

In Figure 3.4, an example outline is shown for a Verification Plan that is based on a standard format for such plans published by the Institute for Electrical and Electronics Engineers (IEEE), Inc.[4]

Engineering SOPs

For the design and building of critical software applications and computerized systems, it is important to have standard operating procedures (SOPs) for software and related hardware engineering activities. When new staff members join the project or temporary programmers are engaged to assist in the development, it is important that they be able to study coding standards and other engineering practices in SOPs so that they can quickly begin work that is consistent and compatible with the rest of the project activities. After the system is built, these same SOPs can help future support personnel in their efforts to repair and modify the system.

Examples for some types of information that should be found in engineering SOPs are given below:

- Conventions for assigning file names (not the names of one's cousins or uncles)

- Rules for interface paths to databases, operating systems, or other platform components, such a file servers, network protocols, analog-to-digital (A/D) converters, or programmable logic controllers (PLCs)

- Consistent language for error messages, help messages, and common screen prompts

---

4. IEEE Standard for Software Verification and Validation Plans—Std. 1012-1986 (The Institute for Electrical and Electronics Engineers, Inc., Piscataway, NJ, 1986), p. 12.

44   The Survive and Thrive Guide to Computer Validation

Figure 3.4. Verification Plan outline (adapted from IEEE Std. 1012-1986)

1. Purpose and scope—Inclusions, exclusions, and limitations

2. Reference documents—SOPs, engineering manuals, policies, and coding standards referenced by this Plan

3. Definitions—Terms required to understand the Verification Plan

4. Verification overview:
   - organization and master schedule for verification effort
   - resources summary and responsibilities for verification tasks
   - tools, techniques, and methodologies used in verification effort

5. SDLC verification tasks:
   - Design Phase—SDD traceability to URS, design interface analysis, design evaluation, and Test Plan development
   - Build Phase—Source code traceability analysis, code evaluation, code interface analysis, source code documentation evaluation, and execution of component and unit testing
   - Test Phase—Execute integration tests, system tests, acceptance tests; write Test Summary Report

6. System verification reporting—Required and optional records and reports to be written and included as package items, including Verification Summary Report

7. Verification administration procedures
   - SDLC problem reporting and resolution process
   - task repeat policy—when and how to repeat tests and other tasks
   - deviation policy—how to handle actions that differ from this Plan
   - control procedures—how system and software are configured, protected, and stored
   - standards, practices, and conventions for verification work—engineering standards, coding conventions, and formats for *verification package* items

---

- Consistent placement of data fields on screens using graphical user interfaces (GUIs)
- Type, format, and extent of technical information to be documented for units of code
- Type, format, and extent of user documentation to be written for the system

- Standard format and content for a system design description (SDD) and required engineering reports

- Testing practices for programmer self-test of code, peer review of code, code walk-throughs, subunit and unit testing, interface testing, integration testing, full-system testing, traceability testing, and acceptance testing

Suppliers can reduce project level rework by having a set of general operating procedures (GOPs) for common items such as engineering reports and testing practices that can be referenced and/or adapted to the needs of a system project.

Configuration Management Logs

Change Control Log

The development of software applications and computerized systems is very sensitive to any changes in the hardware or software components being used in the project. It is important, therefore, to keep a close "change control" record of version and part numbers for all hardware and software components and tools used in the engineering effort during the SDLC of a new system.

The change control record should note a reason for and authorization of a hardware or software change because there are consequences to be considered with such changes. An upgrade to the version of database being used could require changing the standards for calling the database in the application. Introducing a new or updated version of user interface during the project could require reworking all screen files to keep prompts and data fields looking the same on the screen.

Code Management System

It is also very important to manage the changes in the system under development so that when a programmer goes to work on a piece of code, he or she knows that the code being worked on is the latest version being developed. An engineering support tool, such as a code management system, can act as a librarian for the software by providing a secure repository for the developing code and issuing version control identification for each segment of code checked in or out of the repository during development.

Using an automated tool for code management is essential to the success of critical software development projects and makes the SDLC configuration management of system code an achievable objective. It also saves time and money by eliminating confusion, duplication of effort, and rework of code due to the out-of-sequence retrieval of past versions of code, or by having two programmers try to write updates to the same segment of code at the same time. It contributes to the verification of the new system by providing traceability of the system code throughout its SDLC.

Support and Service Logs and Problem Resolution

Records should be kept for support and service activities performed on all hardware and software items used in the SDLC effort. This is usually done by keeping one logbook for the software engineering environment and another logbook for the platform systems supporting the project effort.

A documented process for problem logging and corrective action is also included in this area because a problem often initiates the request for support or service activities. Tracking problems over time can show trends and suggest areas of vulnerability in the system being developed or the platform supporting the project.

System Design Description (SDD)

As discussed in Chapter 2, the SDD document defines the structural blueprint for *how* to build a system to perform the functions described in the user requirements specification (URS). The SDD becomes the common standard for the supplier's engineering team to use in their work of building the system and also in testing the system. It translates the user requirements into a description of software structure, software components, interfaces, and data elements necessary for the system to be built.

For building regulated systems, each user requirement must be traceable to one or more design entities in the SDD and then to one or more coded functions of the completed system that operate to perform that requirement. One part of verification testing includes checking the traceability of the code for critical system functions back to SDD and URS requirements. Keeping the trail clearly identified along the way will make this analysis much easier to perform. It will also help the *owner* and *system team* with regulatory audits at a later date. Sometimes, inspectors ask for records of validation testing that show traceability of critical functions back to the URS.

Further study of the details of software design descriptions can be found in the IEEE *Recommended Practice for Software Design Descriptions* (Std. 1016-1987)[5] and IEEE *Guide to Software Design Descriptions* (Std. 1016.1-1993).[6]

Development Documentation

The type and amount of documents produced during the SDLC will be determined by the engineering SOPs for the project and the supplier's QA organization. Since it is a given fact that many important documents will be produced, it is wise for technical management to establish a document control function for managing critical documentation in a responsible fashion suitable to pass audits and inspections. Some of the types of documents to be cared for include the following:

- Official, signed copy of the URS and any updates or revisions to the URS

- Official, signed copy of the SDD and any updates or revisions to the SDD

- Approved and signed copy of all input and output decision documents for specific system modules in the design-and-build process

---

5. IEEE Recommended Practice for Software Design Descriptions—Std. 1016-1987 (The Institute for Electrical and Electronics Engineers, Inc. Piscataway, NJ, 1986), pp. 1–16.

6. IEEE Guide to Software Design Descriptions—Std. 1016.1-1993 (The Institute for Electrical and Electronics Engineers, Inc. Piscataway, NJ, 1986), pp. 1–22.

48   The Survive and Thrive Guide to Computer Validation

- Official copy of documented code for completed parts of the system
- Approved and signed copy of all engineering SOPs for the project
- Official, signed copy of Verification Plan, Quality Plan, and Audit Reports
- Approved and signed copy of Test Plans, testing documentation and Test Summary Report(s)
- Minutes from joint review meetings with purchaser's representative and supplier's representative

In essence, it is important to archive and control any documents or records of critical decisions made about the design, building, or testing of the system during its SDLC. Final arbiters of what to keep in the way of documentation will be the supplier's QA Unit, technical management, and the Verification Plan.

Quality Plan and Supplier Self-Audit Reports

The supplier should have a documented quality system that is integrated into its whole development process, so that product quality is built-in as development progresses, not "discovered" at the end. The supplier should prepare a Quality Plan for each system development project that describes how its quality system will be applied to the specific project. This would also include a definition of roles and responsibilities, the documentation to be produced for QC activities within the project team, and QA activities outside of the project team for the SDLC of the project.

The Quality Plan should include quality objectives, expressed in measurable terms whenever possible, such as defined input and output criteria for each phase of development. It should define specific responsibilities for quality activities such as reviews and audits, configuration management and change control, and defect control and corrective action.

One important element in the Quality Plan is the scheduling of periodic QA audits of project activities to be sure that the SDD, plans, SOPs, and quality standards are being followed and that quality activities are being performed and adequately documented. The results of audits by the supplier's own QA organization should be written in Self-Audit Reports that are discussed with personnel having responsibility for the audited area. Then a documented procedure for corrective action should be followed by management for any deficiencies found in the audits.

The actual content of Audit Reports is normally considered confidential by a supplier and not open to review by external auditors. Instead, a signed log sheet is kept per audit that identifies who performed the audit, the date of the audit, what area was audited, and the responsible manager receiving the Audit Report. Likewise, a log sheet is completed by the manager and auditor to acknowledge that as of a certain date, appropriate follow-up work was performed to address the deficiencies identified in the audit. Such a traceable record of self-audit and corrective action activity should be sufficient for *owner* and *system team* review unless gross negligence and serious legal harm is at issue due to system failure. In the latter case, legal representatives can subpoena the audit files for examination of their contents.

Verification Testing

The question to be answered by verification testing is, "**Has the software been built right?**" In order to answer this question, testers need to have documented evidence for what "built right" means so that they can write test scripts or cases to challenge the system for its "built right" characteristics. Within the SDLC process, it is the system design description that defines the structural characteristics of "built right." The SDD includes the structural definition of "built right" functions traceable to the URS.

In addition to testing backwards to the SDD, "built right" testing must look forward to examine the "built right" status of technical and user documentation for the new system and the adequacy of any training materials and support plan produced for the system as per Figure 3.5. Do

Figure 3.5. Supplier's verification testing

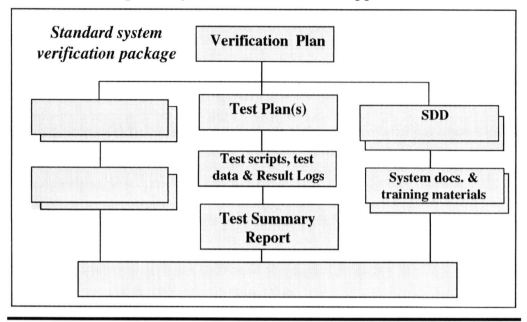

these documents reflect how the system actually operates and what really appears on the screen or printout for a given action or input?

System Documents

There are at least two types of system documents to be checked. One set is for the installation and technical support of the system at the customer site, and one set is for helping the user to operate the system properly. Such documents need to be reviewed for readability and comprehension by their intended audience. The use of technical and nontechnical language must be appropriate to the reader, and the content must be accurate to the state of the system.

Illustrations showing screen displays should be checked for their correlation to actual screens on the system. User

The Supplier's Verification Package **51**

instructions should be read and executed by nonproject personnel to test their clarity, accuracy, and level of detail. Local language translations may have to be planned for certain markets.

Training Materials and Support Plan

An important part of supporting a new system is having useful training materials available for teaching new users how to operate the system. For large systems, this is often a combination of online help and tutorial programs as well as instruction manuals and instructor-taught courses. The various media need to be examined for their accuracy, relevance to the intended audience, and educational effectiveness.

Other elements of the Support Plan must provide for the following:

- System production and corrective action for nonconforming product
- Delivery and installation of the system
- A customer complaint and problem-resolution process
- Product maintenance for problem resolution, interface modifications, functional expansion, or performance improvement
- Release procedures for fixes, upgrades, and new versions of the system

Test Plan(s)

For the SDLC of a large critical system, there will be many Test Plans written and executed at various levels of system design. In order of rising levels of complexity, there will be testing executed at module level, program level, subsystem level, and system level. The strategy for such testing is documented in a Test Plan. Two IEEE definitions for Test Plan and testing are given in Figure 3.6.[7]

---

7. IEEE Standard Glossary of Software Engineering Terminology—Std. 610.12-1990 (The Institute for Electrical and Electronics Engineers, Inc. Piscataway, NJ, 1986), pp. 75–76.

52   The Survive and Thrive Guide to Computer Validation

Figure 3.6. IEEE Glossary of Software Terminology: Std. 610.12-1990

Test plan.

1) A document describing the scope, approach, resources, and schedule of intended test activities. It identifies test items, the features to be tested, the testing tasks, who will do each task, and any risks requiring contingency planning.

2) A document that describes the technical and mechanical approach to be followed for testing a system or component. Typical contents identify the items to be tested, tasks to be performed, responsibilities, schedules, and required resources for the testing activity.

Testing.

1) The process of operating a system or component under specified condition, observing or recording the results, and making an evaluation of some aspect of the system or component.

2) The process of analyzing a software item to detect the differences between existing and required conditions (that is, bugs) and to evaluate the features of the software items.

Test Scripts, Test Data, and Result Logs

While test plans describe the strategy for *what* testing will be done and *what* documentation will be produced, test scripts are written to describe specifically *how* to test a particular item, and result logs record *how* the system has responded to the input of test data designed to challenge its critical functions and characteristics.

Test Data

Test data includes a set of inputs, execution conditions, and expected outputs. Test data are designed to exercise a particular program path or verify compliance with a specific requirement and are associated with one or more test scripts. A set of normal test data might be associated with all or many test scripts, while various sets of problem test data may be associated with a single or a few special focus test scripts. It is important to use both normal and problem or stress test data to challenge a system.

The Supplier's Verification Package   53

Test Scripts

A test script is the same as a test procedure and is a written set of detailed instructions for the setup, execution, and evaluation of results for a given set of test data. The same test script might be used to run both normal and problem test data, but the expected results would obviously be different, and the pass/fail criteria would reflect the test data used.

Result Logs

The Result Log or Test Log is a chronological record of all relevant details about the execution of a test script. It is the document a tester uses to record all system responses and output to test data and test script activity. A Result Log must have an identification that ties it to the respective test script(s) and test data associated with its recorded results.

The log includes a record of any unexpected event occurring that has an impact on the performance of the test or the response of the system, such as loss of power, mechanical failure, or damage to the media containing the test data. It also has a record of any action taken to resolve the unexpected event and the conditions for resuming the testing. Most importantly, it has a test pass/fail statement recorded with the date and signature of the tester performing the test script and making entries in the log.

In addition, the signature and date of a witness to the testing activity are also provided. This witness can be the tester's supervisor or other professional who understands the testing process and verifies that the test was performed and recorded with professional integrity. The witness does not have to stand over the tester all the time, but should make sure at the start of testing that all necessary materials are available, and that the tester understands the test script instructions. After testing is finished, a review of the Result Log for legibility and completeness, and the attachment of any hard copy output required, is sufficient to have the witness sign the log.

Test Summary Report

The Test Summary Report is a document that summarizes testing activities and results and includes an evaluation of the corresponding test items. At the very least, there should be one Test Summary Report for every Test Plan. Depending on the size, scope, and volume of testing being performed, there may be other logical groupings of test scripts and logs to be included in Summary Reports on a program, module, subsystem, or system level.

The Test Summary Report closes the loop that began with the Test Plan. It documents how testing activities and Result Logs challenged the system, and how the system responded for specific objectives stated in the plan. If Result Logs show that the system responded as intended to its challenges and passed any other pass/fail criteria stated in the Test Plan, then the Test Summary Report makes a final evaluation statement, passing the system out of its Testing Phase in the SDLC.

Verification Summary Report

The Verification Summary Report examines all the content of the *verification package* from the perspective of the Verification Plan (Figure 3.7). It provides an overview and analysis of all the verification activities performed and the results of these activities. It summarizes critical difficulties arising and their resolution and makes an assessment of system quality based upon the Test Summary Report and other package items.

Finally, the Verification Summary Report makes a recommendation about the status of the system. On the basis of review and analysis, an evaluation of the system is made, and a release statement is decided and signed. There are three types of system release statements that can be made:

- Full release of the entire system for customer shipment without reservation

- Partial release of the system due to specific modules being incomplete or some other reason that limits it use

Figure 3.7. Validation Summary Report

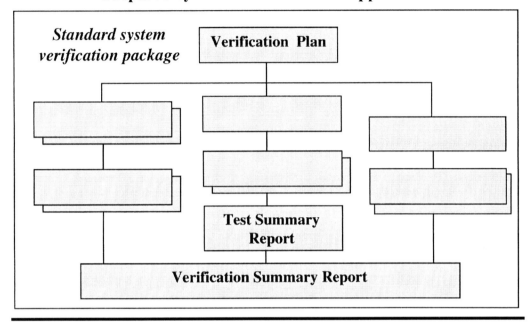

- Release denied due to lack of critical system elements, deficiencies in *verification package* items, or failure of the system to pass Testing Phase

III. Conclusion

System Quality Must Be Planned, Built-in, and Documented, Not Discovered

The development of critical software applications and computerized systems for regulated environments requires that rigorous quality practices be applied by the supplier throughout the SDLC. A casual approach to software development is not allowed, and the process of building quality into the system must be supported by documented evidence, such as that found in a supplier's *verification package* (Figure 3.2). External suppliers for whom systems development is a full-time business are often better

56   The Survive and Thrive Guide to Computer Validation

equipped to support the quality infrastructure required for building large, critical systems to regulated standards. The purchase decision for a critical system is an important one, and *system sponsors, owners,* and *system teams* can use this discussion of the *verification package* to help them evaluate the ability of various suppliers to support their computer validation needs.

4. The Owner's Validation Package

I. System Sponsor's Summary

The purchase, installation, and use of critical software applications and computerized systems for handling regulated data or controlling regulated processes requires the development of an *owner's validation package*. The *validation package* provides documented evidence of the quality of the system throughout its whole life cycle as per Figure 4.1. This includes all the activities for which the *sponsor* and *owner* are directly responsible plus audits of the supplier's *verification package* for the system development life cycle (SDLC).

It is the *system sponsor's* responsibility to give final approval of the *validation package* and signatory release of the system for use as a validated system in regulated activities. This process is initiated by the *owner* and *system team* preparing a system's Validation Plan for the *Sponsor's* review and approval.

After the Validation Plan has been approved by the *sponsor*, it is implemented by the *system team*. A standard body of documented evidence is built into a *validation package* (see Figure 4.2). The whole package is then reviewed and analyzed by the *Owner* in a Summary Validation Report that includes a recommended release status. The *sponsor's* review and signatory approval of the Validation Summary Report affirms the validation status of the system and releases it for regulated use.

57

58   The Survive and Thrive Guide to Computer Validation

Figure 4.1. System owner's validation focus

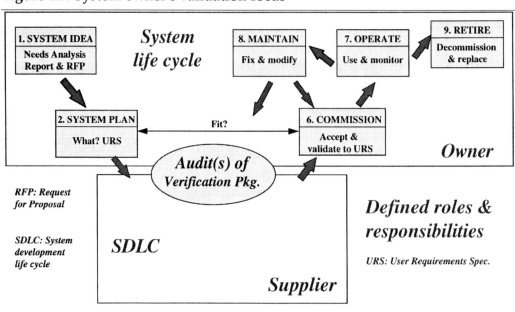

Figure 4.2. System owner's validation package

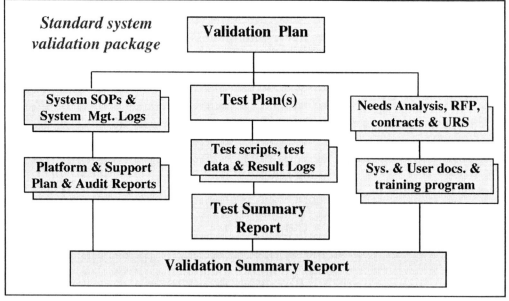

On a periodic basis, updates to the Summary Validation Report will be made by the *owner* to reflect changes and modifications made to the system and to items in the *validation package*. The *sponsor*'s review and approval of these updates keeps the release status of the system current and shows due diligence on the part of management for maintaining the validation status of the system.

II. System Owner and System Team Discussion

The three major objectives of the *system owner* and *system team* are to ensure that the system

1. is under control, ready and available for users,

2. performs its intended functions in a reliable manner, and

3. protects and maintains the integrity of the data it handles and/or the process it controls.

For systems operating in regulated activities, a fourth objective is to provide documented evidence of system quality so that the system can pass inspections by outside authorities without incurring major criticism. Actually, when a review is made of all the various computer regulations around the world, every item in their content can be classified under one of these four themes—management control, data integrity, system reliability, and auditable quality.

The items shown in the standard validation package of Figure 4.2 are evidence of the good practice activities required to ensure that a strategic system works well over time and gives a positive return on investment (ROI) for its purchase. Preparing and maintaining such a standard package gives the *sponsor*, QA auditor, and other management people an objective view of the quality of the system's contribution to the business process it supports. The various plans, logs, and reports clearly define the amount of time and resource required to manage the system; this supports a more realistic budgeting process for maintaining such systems in a validated state.

Owner's Validation Plan

In an ideal world, the *system sponsor, owner,* and *system team* are assigned their roles and prepare the first draft of the system's Validation Plan as part of the needs analysis process. The *owner* and *system team* participate actively in the preparation of the request for proposal (RFP) and the supplier selection and contracting process (Figure 4.3). It is important that any specific regulations for computer validation required by the business process be included in the RFP and that the chosen supplier (internal or external) understands such regulations and agrees to abide by them in the SDLC process.

The Validation Plan document is prepared by the *system owner* and *system team* and then reviewed and approved by the *system sponsor*. It is intended to be a prospective plan for how to ensure quality throughout all the phases of a

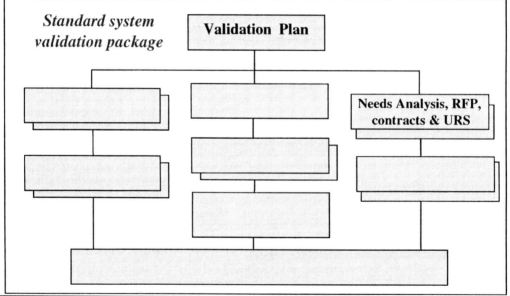

Figure 4.3. Owner's Validation Plan

system's life cycle from initial planning and development to ultimate retirement and replacement. Common sense dictates that there will be several versions of and/or updates to the Validation Plan over the life of the system. It is important that change control be closely kept for this document and that the *sponsor* review and sign approval of each new version or update to the Plan prior to the implementation of its content by the *owner* and *system team*.

Experience has shown that it is useful to reference the Institute for Electrical and Electronics Engineers (IEEE), Inc. Standard for Software Verification and Validation Plans and adapt it to the size and scope of the system being validated.[1] Usually, the SDLC phases are covered by auditing the supplier and reviewing the supplier's verification package. The major focus of the Validation Plan concentrates on the *owner's* role in system planning, developing user requirements specification (URS), and the remaining non-SDLC phases of the total life cycle as per Figure 4.1.

The following example of a System Validation Plan outline is adapted from the IEEE Std. 1012-1986 (Figure 4.4). This standard, along with many other useful standards, can be found in the IEEE Standards Collection for Software Engineering which is an essential reference volume for any *system team*.[2]

In order to make the work more manageable, the Validation Plan usually divides the computerized system into two components: a software application designed to perform a regulated function and a platform system which includes all other software, hardware and network components required to enable the application to perform its intended function in the business process (Figure 1.4). The software application is a definite "inclusion" for the Validation Plan and is the primary focus for all package items.

---

1. IEEE Standard for Software Verification and Validation Plans—Std. 1012-1986 (The Institute for Electrical and Electronics Engineers, Inc., Piscataway, NJ, 1986), p. 12.

2. IEEE Standards Collection: Software Engineering (The Institute for Electrical and Electronics Engineers, Inc., Piscataway, NJ, 1994).

62   The Survive and Thrive Guide to Computer Validation

Figure 4.4. Validation Plan outline (adapted from IEEE Std. 1012-1986)

1. Purpose and scope—Inclusions, exclusions and limitations

2. Reference documents—SOPs, manuals, and policies referenced by the Plan

3. Definitions—Terms required to understand the Validation Plan

4. Validation overview

   - organization and master schedule for the validation effort

   - resources summary and responsibilities for validation tasks

   - tools, techniques, and methodologies used in the validation effort

5. Life cycle validation tasks—From purchase/install to retirement

   - Concept Phase—Needs Analysis, RFP, and URS

   - Development Phase—QA Audit Reports of supplier(s)

   - Installation and Checkout Phase—Test and Validation Summary Reports

   - Operation and Maintenance Phase—SOPs, logs, audits, and training

   - Retirement Phase—Archive Plan and Transition Plan to next system

6. System validation reporting—Required and optional records/reports to be written

7. Validation administration procedures

   - reporting and resolution process for system and user problems and issues

   - task repetition policy—when and how to repeat testing and other validation tasks

   - deviation policy—how to handle actions that differ from the Plan

   - control procedures—how software application and platform system(s) are configured, protected, and stored

   - standards, practices, and conventions for validation work—template formats for logs, reports, and other items in the validation package

---

The platform system, as a configured group of items, is covered under a "limitations" section of the Validation Plan with the platform supplier providing a separate validation effort and platform package as part of a support plan with the *owner*. The internals of individual software and hardware components of the platform system are

The Owner's Validation Package   63

considered "exclusions" for both the application and platform validation packages. They are quality checked only for their performance as a configured platform in enabling the application to operate as intended. When the application passes its validation testing, the configured platform components are considered to be of sufficient quality to allow the application to do its work and are not tested further on their own.

When the database software on a platform system allows an application to operate its functions for retrieval and data handling as intended, the database software itself does not become the subject of further testing. The practical limit for the Validation Plan of a software application rests with that application being shown to work as intended in its operating environment, and, with the components of a platform system, being able to work as a platform unit configured to properly support the application in performing its work. For the purposes of the Validation Plan, testing for the application will provide "black box" testing of the platform system and its components.

Validation Testing

In Chapter 3, it stated that the question to be answered by the supplier's verification testing is, "**Has the software been built right?**" and structural or "white box" testing is performed against technical functions traceable to the system design description (SDD). Here, in the *owner's* area of validation testing, the question to be answered is, "**Has the right software been built?**" and functional or "black box" testing is performed against business requirements traceable to the user requirements specification (URS).

If the business process or data handling characteristics have changed greatly, and the URS has not been updated, it could well be that the software may have been "built right" but may no longer be the "right software" for the *owner's* changed situation. One of the advantages to developing the Validation Plan early in the system idea and planning process is that version control of the URS would be required, and the URS would be kept up-to-date with significant changes in the business process. The purchaser's representative would then communicate such changes to the supplier so that the SDD could also be kept current, and the "right software" would be "built right."

The opportunity for wrong software being built right is often likely to occur with internal suppliers, where less formal RFP, URS, and contractual relations usually exist. Often people assume that others in their same company know of changes in their department and do not think to document the changes or their impact on other activities outside the department. This is one instance where formal computer validation practices can help a company avoid costly mistakes with the development of internal service level agreements (ISLAs) for software projects managed by representatives from both departments.

Validation Test Plan(s)

A Validation Test Plan is the document that sets forth the strategy for examining, stressing, and analyzing the system for its ability to perform as intended by the URS under normal and problem conditions found in the *owner's* operating environment. The *system owner* and *system team* develop the Test Plan with a focus on the normally acceptable limits of performance, as well as the usual out of bounds and problem situations likely to occur in the working environment. The goal is not to break the system or push it into disaster mode, but to give it some heavy-duty stressing that the rigors of unexpected workload and the misadventures of inexperienced staff can sometimes produce.

For very large, complex systems, there may be one Master Test Plan that defines a number of specialized test plans to be prepared to focus on individual modules of the system used in different departments and on the critical internal and external interfaces of the system. Each plan will describe the scope, approach, resources, and schedule of intended activities. It will identify test items, features to be tested, features not to be tested and why, the testing tasks,

The Owner's Validation Package   65

who performs each task, and any risks requiring contingency planning. Figure 4.5 shows an example of a Test Plan outline adapted from the IEEE Standard for Software Test Documentation.[3]

Figure 4.5. Test Plan outline (adapted from IEEE Std. 829-1983)

1. Test Plan ID number—Coded to relate to the associated Validation Plan

2. Introduction—Items to be tested and reference to related URS

3. Test items—List of software applications and system versions to be tested

4. Features to be tested

5. Features not to be tested and why (installed feature not used by the application)

6. Approach—Describes overall strategy, techniques and limits for testing

    • traceability analysis of system functions to URS

    • use of system and user documentation in test scripts

    • risk analysis to define primary focus for testing activities—IQ/OQ/PQ

    • interface testing with systems A, B, and C . . . on the network

7. Item pass/fail criteria—If one test script fails, does whole system fail?

8. Testing suspension criteria and resumption requirements

9. Test deliverables—Documents required: Test Plan, Test Cases, Test Logs, Test Summary Report (templates included in appendices)

10. Testing tasks—Tasks necessary to prepare for, execute, and report testing

11. Environmental needs—Physical, logical, and security requirements for testing

12. Responsibilities—Identified for test developer, tester, and witness

13. Staff training needs—Specify skill level for test writer, tester, and witness

14. Schedule—Estimated time to do each task and define milestones

15. Risks and contingencies—Identify high-risk assumptions of Test Plan and specify backup plan to support each

16. Approvals—Specify names and titles of all who must approve this Plan, with space for signatures and dates

---

3. IEEE Standard for Software Test Documentation—Std. 829-1983 (The Institute for Electrical and Electronics Engineers, Inc., Piscataway, NJ, 1993), p. 10.

Test Scripts, Test Data, and Result Logs

In order for the *owner's* validation testing to be auditable, it must be fully documented as per Figure 4.6. Testing performed without proper documentation is considered not to have been done by auditors and inspectors. Having a written Test Plan is the first step, but this must be followed by test scripts to give instructions for the test, test data for both normal and problem situations, and logs for recording results and observations made during tests. Test scripts are usually executed by the system users because they are in the best position to assess the system's fit to the work process, or "right software" testing.

In order to make this testing process more practical and more profitable, it is good to use, as much as possible, the instructions and descriptions in the system and user documentation as part of the test scripts. These reduce copying procedures in the scripts and allow for checking to see if the system and user documents are written clearly, and if

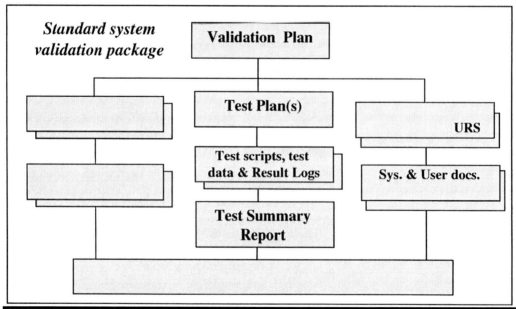

Figure 4.6. Owner's validation testing

The Owner's Validation Package   67

they accurately reflect the way the system operates. It also trains the user testers in the content and usefulness of the system documentation.

An example of a test script and a Test Log is given in Figure 4.7. These are not meant to be taken as absolutes, but are just given as one illustration of the process of

---

Figure 4.7. Test Script & Result Log outline (adapted from IEEE Std. 829-1983)

Test Script

1.   Test script identifier: Relates it to the associated Test Plan and identifies script author.

2.   Purpose: What feature or function is this script testing? Reference system documentation for description of feature or function.

3.   Special requirements: List special equipment, tester training, or input materials needed.

4.   Test procedure steps: Specific instructions to the tester—Refer to system and user manuals or SOPs for description of specific tasks.

5.   Specify use of Result Log and identify type of output to be collected-screen printouts, reports, graphs, etc. Provide a listing of expected output for steps in the test procedure.

6.   Provide a set of test data for both normal and problem situations.

Result Log

1.   Testing Log: (Identifier relates it to associated test script.)
     - space identified for recording observed results from specific steps in the test procedure

2.   Unexpected events occurring:
     - space to record any problem or issue arising during testing

3.   Resolution of unexpected events:
     - space to record problem or issue resolution

4.   Acceptance Criteria—Should apply Test Plan criteria

5.   Conclusion statement on system status—System passed/failed test script

6.   Tester signature and date

7.   Witness signature and date

68   The Survive and Thrive Guide to Computer Validation

documenting test procedures and logging the results. The items included are important, but their format and detail are up to the scope of the system being tested. One critical factor is that the author of the test script should *never* be the person executing it as tester. The script author may, however, be a witness to the testing and sign the Result Log in the capacity of witness.

When testing is performed in regulated environments, it is important that testers understand the kind of practices which are required for their work to be accepted by auditors and inspectors. A set of common good testing practices is given in Figure 4.8.

Figure 4.8. The do's and don'ts of testing regulated systems

Do:

1. Do carefully read through test script, test data, and Result Log before starting test procedure.

2. Do check testing area to be sure that all materials required for testing are present such as access privileges to test database, printers and diskettes to output test results as needed, and scheduled system time to perform the testing activities.

3. Do explain testing process to the witness and execute first test script.

4. Do use ONLY a ballpoint pen to record any results in the Result Log. Print words in block letters for clearer reading of results. Write "Okay" or "OK" for an affirmative answer instead of a check mark and "Yes" or "No" instead of "Y" or "N."

5. Do correct a mistake with the following procedure:

    • Draw a single line through the result so that it is still visible.

    • Write in the new result beside the lined out item.

    • Initial and date the time of correction.

    • Explain why the correction was made if the reason is not intuitively obvious.

Continued on next page.

The Owner's Validation Package   69

Continued from previous page.

6. Do complete all items in the Result Log corresponding to each test script. When there are large open spaces in the results area, draw a line through the space or down the rest of the blank page to show that no more result information is to be recorded there.

7. Do record any unexpected event that occurs to disrupt the testing process, such as power failure, disk crash, or coffee spilled on keyboard. Record any deviation from the system view and the testing materials provided, such as typos in test script when describing screen views.

8. Do sign and date all printouts requested by the test script.

9. Do sign and date any diskette of result files requested by the test script.

10. Do bring all materials to witness at the end of testing. Review the package items with the witness to explain how the testing was performed and results were logged, as well as what printouts or diskette files were prepared as records of test output.

Don't:

1. Don't use pencil or any other erasable medium to record test results.

2. Don't use correction fluid or any other erasing material to remove recorded results or correct them.

3. Don't use checkmarks, ditto marks, "Y/N" or other abbreviations when recording results. Write out results and comments in full.

4. Don't leave large blank spaces on the Results Log. Draw a line down the rest of the page or blank space to show that nothing more is to be added to the result.

5. Don't forget to sign and date all output documents and logs.

Test Summary Report

After all the test scripts have been executed, the *system owner* works with the IT person on the *system team* to write the Test Summary Report (Figure 4.9). This document reviews all of the activities performed under the Test Plan, analyzes the handling of any unexpected problems or issues arising, and provides an evaluation of the system

70 The Survive and Thrive Guide to Computer Validation

Figure 4.9. Test Summary Report (adapted from IEEE Std. 829-1983)

1. Report identifier: Reference number related to associated Test Plan

2. Summary of activities: Identifies items tested, testing environment, and resources applied

3. Variances: Summary of deviations from Test Plan and rationale for deviations

4. Summary of results: Summarizes results from all test scripts and identifies both resolved and unresolved problems and issues arising

5. Evaluation: Overall assessment of each tested item based upon Result Logs and pass/fail criteria

6. Suitability Assessment: Conclusion statement on system's suitability for work based upon the Test Plan criteria

7. Approvals: Owner, IT, and QC signatures & dates

based on Result Logs and the pass/fail criteria of the Test Plan.

Owners often find it useful to have three levels of pass/fail evaluation when working with large, complex systems. The levels would be full pass, provisional pass, and fail. The provisional pass category allows the system to be used within the limits of certain stated provisions such as various independent modules being used even though some other parts of the system have not been tested yet or another type of restriction applies to prevent a full pass grade. It is important that a rationale for the provisional pass be included in the Suitability Assessment of the Test Summary Report.

Commission Phase Testing—Acceptance, IQ, OQ, PQ

During the process of commissioning a new system into a regulated environment, there are two types of testing performed: acceptance testing and qualification testing. Acceptance testing is formal testing conducted to determine

The Owner's Validation Package   71

whether or not a system satisfies its acceptance criteria (as per contract or URS) and to enable the customer to determine whether or not to accept the system. Qualification testing is testing conducted to determine whether a system or component is suitable for operational use.

Within qualification testing, there are three themes of concern that need to be addressed and are defined below.[4] These may be tested by separate sets of test scripts or by any combination of test scripts which challenge the system for their respective concerns.

1. *Installation Qualification (IQ):* Documented verification that all key aspects of the installation adhere to approved design intentions according to system specifications and that manufacturers' recommendations are suitably considered.

2. *Operational Qualification (OQ):* Documented verification that each unit or subsystem operates as intended throughout its anticipated operating range.

3. *Performance Qualification (PQ):* Documented verification that the integrated system performs as intended in its normal operating environment.

Usually IQ and some level of OQ are included in acceptance testing, which also checks for other contractual requirements of the supplier having been met. A more specific, process-dependent OQ and full PQ focus is included in the validation testing, which also looks to stress the system in its working environment.

Operation Phase Validation

While it is quite normal for the *system owner* and *system team* to put a large focus on various testing activities for a new system, it is important to remember that for a validated system to pass audits and inspections, there must be

---

4. T. Stokes, R.C. Branning, K.G. Chapman, et al., *Good Computer Validation Practices: Common Sense Implementation* (Interpharm Press, Inc., Buffalo Grove, IL, 1994), p. 281.

72   The Survive and Thrive Guide to Computer Validation

a documented configuration management environment to keep the system working properly. The items shown in Figure 4.10 provide such an environment.

The activities represented by these documents continue as ongoing support for the system throughout its operational phase. Edits and updates are made in a controlled way to reflect changes in the system and working environment, and the reliability of the system is closely monitored and maintained in a predictable manner until its retirement.

System Standard Operating Procedures (SOPs)

For both the software application and the platform system, inspectors will expect to see a basic set of SOPs that describe the appropriate way for users and support personnel to work with the system. If more than one validated

Figure 4.10. Operation phase validation

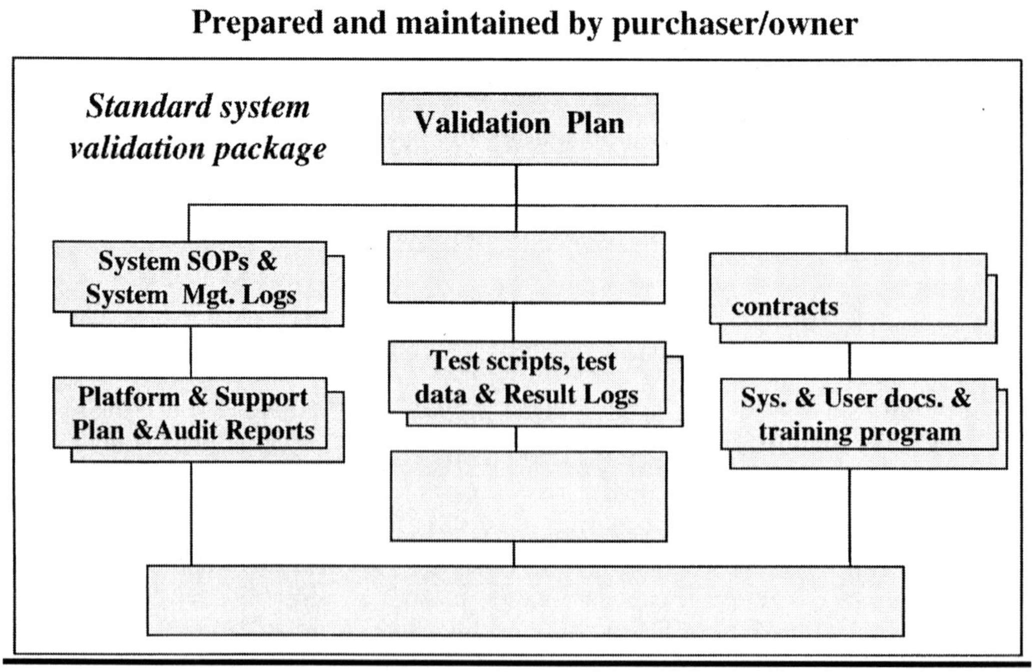

Prepared and maintained by purchaser/owner

Standard system validation package

Validation Plan

System SOPs & System Mgt. Logs

contracts

Platform & Support Plan & Audit Reports

Test scripts, test data & Result Logs

Sys. & User docs. & training program

application is hosted on the same platform system, a single set of SOPs can serve the platform. An SOP per application can then note the specific differences or additions from the basic set that are required for the special needs of individual applications, such as time and frequency for data backup.

In April 1995, the Organization for Economic Cooperation and Development (OECD) published a GLP Consensus Document for computerized systems used in laboratories. This document gave a recommended list of core SOPs for the good practice of regulated systems that is shown in Figure 4.11.[5] The *system owner* and the *system team* would be wise to ensure that such a set of SOPs was put in place for their computerized system.

Figure 4.11. Basic set of standard operating procedures (SOPs) (OECD GLP Consensus: Section 8)

Procedures for:

1. Operation of computerized systems (hardware/software), and the responsibilities of personnel involved

2. Security measures used to detect and prevent unauthorized access and program changes

3. Authorization for program changes and the recording of changes

4. Authorization for changes to equipment (hardware/software), including testing before use, if appropriate

5. Periodic testing for correct functioning of the complete system or its component parts and the recording of these tests

6. Maintenance of computerized systems and any associated equipment

7. Software development and acceptance testing and the recording of all acceptance testing

8. Backup of all stored data and contingency plans in the event of a breakdown

9. Archiving and retrieval of all documents, software, and computer data

10. Monitoring and auditing of computerized systems

---

5. *GLP Consensus Document: The Application of the Principles of GLP to Computerized Systems*, Environment Monograph No. 116, (Environment Directorate, OECD, Paris, 1995), Section 8.

System Management Logs

While SOPs tell users and support personnel how to operate and manage the system, documented evidence to prove that SOPs have been followed is found in various System Management Logs. Here, records are made with date and signature for data and system backups, maintenance and calibration activities, problem reports and their resolution, service calls, parts replaced or software patches installed, security authorizations and changes, and all other SOP actions. A *system owner* and *system team* can establish a logical set of logbook records for the system at commissioning; this will integrate evidence of SOP compliance into the normal workflow of the system from the beginning.

Platform and Support Plan and Contracts

It is important to document the configuration of the platform system supporting a regulated software application and to manage that platform under strict change control. Usually, the platform system is provided by a IT organization outside of the *system owner's* area, and validation testing of the platform is performed by this internal IT supplier.

A Validation Team should negotiate a written Support Plan with its IT supplier for the platform system and application. An internal service level agreement (ISLA) can be written to describe the roles and responsibilities of both parties for keeping the application and platform in a validated state. The ISLA should also include any activities required to maintain the integrity of the regulated data handled by the system.

Audit Reports

QA professionals who are separate from any QC professionals participating on the *system team* are expected to perform periodic audits of the system and its validation package items. As with any other audit, they look for documented evidence of compliance to required regulations, policies, SOPs, and plans. The audit should be performed according to an SOP for audits in the QA Department and a written report should be presented to the *system owner* and *sponsor*.

Most companies consider the content of System Audit Reports to be company confidential and not subject to casual review by inspectors. The important issue for an inspector is whether an audit was made and whether any follow-up action was taken. A signature and date record of the auditor's visit should be kept in the System Management Log, as well as a signature and date of the *owner's* receipt of the Audit Report. Later, another signature and date should be made by the *owner* and auditor to acknowledge that follow-up work has been completed for recommendations in the Audit Report.

Ongoing Quality Control Testing and Repeat Validation Testing

The *system owner* and the *system team* should plan for the ongoing use of some validation test scripts as QC test sets for the system. The QC test data should include both problem and stress cases as well as normal range data, so that both the responsiveness and robustness of the system is monitored. Whenever fixes or updates are made to the system, the basic set of QC test data can be updated to reflect the new changes and run again as part of a mini-commissioning process after the change. The use of an automated testing tool can remove the human workload for much of this ongoing QC testing.

System and User Documents and Training Program

When fixes and updates are made to the system, it is important that system manuals, logbooks, user SOPs, and training materials are reviewed for possible changes needed to keep current with how the system operates. It is also important for the *owner* to communicate all changes to the system users and the *system team*; this can be accomplished through the publication of "training notes" by electronic mail that can then be printed out and put into training materials, as well as being stored online in a notes section to the Help file.

The *system owner* and the *system team* need to be sure that a training program is defined for teaching new personnel how to use and support the system. Depending on the complexity of the system, this program can be a mix of on-the-job training by an experienced colleague, formal classes, online help and system training modules, or other self-paced training methods.

Materials appropriate to the style of training need to be ready and available to new users, and their experience with the training must be recorded in a training file. A second element in training is refresher training for users who leave the area and later return to an updated system. When major modifications are made, or a new version of the system is released, training must be planned for all users, and their attendance at such training should be recorded in their training file and the system logbook.

Validation Summary Report

The last step in preparing a *validation package* is the *system owner's* preparation of a Validation Summary Report. This is done after the first commissioning is completed, and updates are made later to the Validation Summary Report as renewed commissioning activities take place following the installation of major modifications and new versions of the system. The Validation Plan itself should state in its Task Repeat Policy how often and under what circumstances an update to the Validation Summary Report is to be made (Figure 4.12).

In the Validation Summary Report, the *system owner* reviews all of the activities performed under the Validation Plan and recorded in various items of the *validation package* and gives a summary of the highlights of the validation

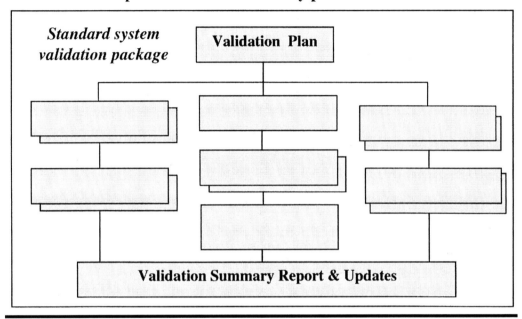

Figure 4.12. Validation Summary Report

effort. Both problems and successes are discussed, and an overall assessment is made of the system's suitability for its intended work. A recommendation is then made for the *sponsor* to release the system for validated use in the business process. An example for the outline of a Validation Summary Report is shown in Figure 4.13.[6]

III. Conclusion

A Standard System Package Supports System Reliability and Inspectability

The *owner's* system *validation package* covers the whole life cycle of the system from concept through retirement. While

---

6. IEEE Standard for Software Verification and Validation Plans—Std. 1012-1986 (The Institute for Electrical and Electronics Engineers, Inc., Piscataway, NJ, 1986), p. 18.

78   The Survive and Thrive Guide to Computer Validation

Figure 4.13. Validation Summary Report (adapted from IEEE Std. 1012-1986)

1. Plan identifier: ID number indicating system associated with the Plan

2. Summary of all validation life cycle tasks

3. Summary of all validation package items and their current status

4. Summary of unexpected problems/issues arising and their resolution

5. Summary of deviations from the Validation Plan and rationale for deviations

6. Assessment of overall system quality based upon the Test Summary Report, Audit Report, and training results

7. Recommendations: Statement from management for the validation status of the target system

8. Approval signature(s) and date(s)

Appendices:

Update Report(s) on major system changes and extensive retesting

Summary Report(s) for periodic quality control testing

---

testing is a major flow of activity in the package effort, there are other important activities under the Validation Plan associated with providing an appropriate operational environment for the system. Testing by itself is not sufficient, and undocumented testing is worthless for audit and inspection purposes.

Developing and maintaining a system's *validation package* is significant work, and the *system sponsor, owner,* and *system team* need to plan for the time and effort required to accomplish it. The return for such effort will be management control of the computerized system, assured integrity of system data handling, reliability of system performance, and documented evidence of system quality for passing audits and inspections.

5. The Retrospective Evaluation Package

I. System Sponsor's Summary

Companies often have strategic software applications and computerized systems that have been working for many years and have never been validated. Such systems are called "legacy systems" by regulatory inspectors. If they are considered critical to a regulated process, documented evidence will be sought to prove their quality. Since the burden of proof for quality comes a long time after purchase and installation, the *sponsor* looks to the *system owner* and *system team* to develop a *retrospective evaluation package* for the legacy system.

The focus of retrospective attention begins with the system's performance in today's working environment and then works its way back through the history of the system to its original purchase. A search is made to collect all relevant documents and a timeline is created based on the documents and other records found (Figure 5.1).

Based on the timeline, the person knowing the most about the system writes a brief history of the validation-relevant issues concerning system performance and reliability over time and ends with a description of how the system is used today. The *system owner* and *system team* prepare a *retrospective evaluation package* (Figure 5.2) and the *sponsor* reviews and signs the Evaluation Summary Report.

The rationale for this retrospective effort is to bring the system under management control with a documented quality

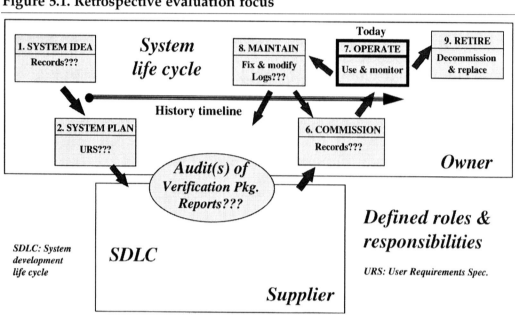

Figure 5.1. Retrospective evaluation focus

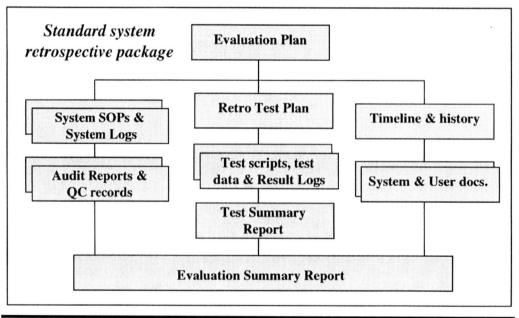

Figure 5.2. Retrospective evaluation package

The Retrospective Evaluation Package   **81**

process so that continued operation of the system will be in compliance with regulatory standards for computer validation. Sometimes, it also happens that through the evaluation process, a clear case is made for replacing the system rather than continuing its use due to quality and reliability issues observed. In such an instance, the *sponsor* can then make an informed decision about investments that will directly impact the quality of the business.

II. System Owner and System Team Discussion

In retrospective work, as in prospective work, the major objectives of the *system owner* and *system team* are to ensure that

- the system is under control, ready and available for users,

- it performs its intended functions in a reliable manner,

- it protects and maintains the integrity of the data it handles and/or the process it controls, and

- that the system has documented evidence of its quality suitable for audit and inspection purposes.

The items shown in the standard retrospective evaluation package of Figure 5.2 are evidence of the good practice activities necessary to ensure that a "due diligence" effort has been made to establish the quality record of a legacy system in the past by a review of timeline documents and history of QC records. The package items also show that the necessary documented quality practices (SOPs, logs, audits, testing, and system and user documentation) are defined and working for the system to function as intended today and in the future. The strategy developed by the *system owner* and *system team* to accomplish the tasks necessary to produce the *retrospective evaluation package* is defined in a written Evaluation Plan for the system. This plan is prepared in much the same way as a Verification or Validation Plan (Figure 5.3).[1]

---

1. IEEE Standard for Software Verification and Validation Plans—Std. 1012-1986 (The Institute for Electrical and Electronics Engineers, Inc., Piscataway, NJ, 1986), p. 12.

82   The Survive and Thrive Guide to Computer Validation

Figure 5.3. Evaluation Plan outline (adapted from IEEE Std. 1012-1986)

1. Purpose and scope—Inclusions, exclusions, and limitations

2. Reference documents—SOPs, manuals, and policies referenced by the Plan

3. Definitions—Terms required to understand the Evaluation Plan

4. Retrospective Evaluation overview
    *   organization and master schedule for the evaluation effort
    *   resources summary and responsibilities for evaluation tasks
    *   tools, techniques, and methodologies used in the evaluation effort

5. Life cycle evaluation review—From purchase/install to present time
    *   Purchase and Development Phase—by timeline and history document
    *   Installation and Checkout Phase—by timeline and history document
    *   Operation and Maintenance Phase—by System Logs and QC records
    *   Present Phase—by Test Plan(s) and documentation review/update

6. System evaluation reporting—Required and optional records/reports to be written

7. Evaluation administration procedures:
    *   system problem/issue reporting and resolution
    *   task repeat policy—when and how to repeat tests and other tasks
    *   deviation policy—handling actions that differ from the Plan
    *   control procedures—how to store, manage, and protect original documents for software application, platform system, and evaluation package
    *   approval process for evaluation package, Summary Reports, and final release status for the system

---

The Evaluation Plan

The validation concerns of an Evaluation Plan are the same as for prospective work. They are management control of the system, integrity of data and data handling on the system, system reliability to perform as intended, and auditable quality. It is only the delayed start of validation work in the system life cycle of the legacy system that gives a different perspective to the documented evidence in an *retrospective evaluation package.*

The most common concern with legacy systems is a lack of organized documentation for the system and its operation over time. Depending on the age of the system, it may be quite a detective effort for the *system team* to find past records pertaining to the system, but a reasonable attempt has to be made to document the system (Figure 5.4).

Timeline and History

Documenting a legacy system begins with collecting any life cycle records pertaining to the system since its first purchase and use in the organization. If an official Needs Analysis was not performed, there may have been some other document prepared to justify the purchase and to identify the user requirements and reasons for acquiring the system. For a software application, some examples of relevant documents would include the following:

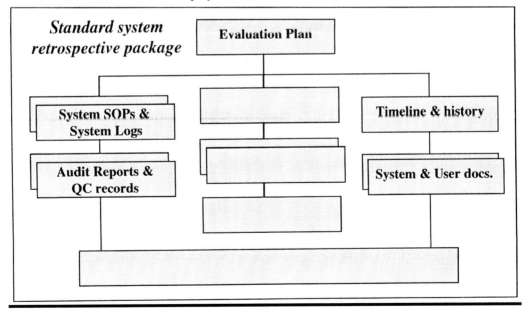

Figure 5.4. Documenting the system

- Request for proposal and purchase order
- Acceptance release form and testing documents
- System SOPs and operating logbooks
- Maintenance and upgrade records and service contracts
- Control Log for code changes, fixes, or new versions
- System and user manuals, user SOPs, training materials, and training records
- Audit Reports of the supplier and ongoing use of the system

Records for the platform system supporting a software application can be more difficult to identify in retrospect when the application is hosted in a large environment with many applications on the same or shared systems. Part of installation and acceptance testing should have included reference to having the appropriate platform components to meet the manufacturer's specifications. Certainly the platform for today can be documented with hardware, software, database, and network configurations. Also, the SOPs for managing the platform today can be included.

In general, relevant documents for platform systems would include the following:

- Service contracts and maintenance and support records
- Vendor product manuals for hardware, software, database, and network components
- System Operating Logs
- Change control records for installation of upgrades and fixes
- SOPs for system management to include backup, recovery, and disaster recovery
- Data archiving SOP
- Physical and logical security policies
- Experience and training records for technical staff supporting the platform

The Retrospective Evaluation Package   85

Timeline

After collecting all available retrospective documentation, a list is written to inventory and organize the documents according to date. This date sequence then establishes a system "timeline" that can be supported by "documented evidence." There is no need for the *system team* to be obsessive about making a timeline that covers every detail, because with legacy systems, there are bound to be holes in the documented evidence. The older the system, the more holes will be found. Creating the timeline does, however, provide an organized approach for reviewing collected evidence, relating it to the life cycle of the legacy system, and supporting the effort to write a history document.

History Document—Yesterday and Today

The system history document has two parts: one addresses the past and one describes the present operation of the legacy system. In the first part, the individual with the most knowledge of the system's past uses the timeline and its documentation to write a summary history of how the system has been used and operated over time. If there is no Needs Analysis Report or User Requirements Specification available in the timeline documentation, the writing of the history document can be used to identify user needs by discussing how the system was operated in the work process.

In the second part of a history document, the individual with the most knowledge of how the system operates today uses current timeline events and documentation to write a Summary Report of recent user experience with the system in its operating environment. This report references diagrams and flowcharts for today's configuration of the system and identifies the owner and key user groups.

Part Two also describes the important user needs for the system and references the quality assurance practices that are in place today to ensure that strategic functions work as intended. It references supplier contracts for service and support and describes system capabilities and recordkeeping logs for backup, disaster recovery, security, and control of change. Finally, training for new users and for updates to the system would be discussed.

86   The Survive and Thrive Guide to Computer Validation

Each author signs and dates his or her respective part of the history document. Along with the signature, a brief description is included that informs the reader of relevant career experience which qualifies the author to write about the legacy system.

System SOPs and System Logs

Legacy systems often lack or have limited sets of formal procedures and written records. It is important that the *owner* and *system team* not try to recreate missing logs and SOPs from past operations, as that would be considered fraud by auditors and inspectors. Equally important, however, is to fill the holes of missing SOPs and log records for today by establishing new SOPs and logbooks for current and future work with the system. In other words, the *system owner* cannot undo past inadequacies, but the *system owner* is expected to establish a properly documented environment for operating the system in compliance with accepted standards for today and tomorrow.

System SOPs

In Figure 5.5, the basic set of OECD SOPs has been applied to the legacy system situation that is essentially the same as for new systems.[2] The methods for ensuring the quality of a computerized system in operation remain the same regardless of the age of the system.

In highly regulated industries, such as pharmaceuticals and biotechnology, every company has its own format for writing SOPs. This is acceptable as long as the SOP clearly communicates the necessary procedures and identifies the roles responsible for such procedures. The exact format is not important, and there is no single standard for SOP documents, but experience has shown than most of the common elements for clear communication are included in the SOP outline shown in Figure 5.6.

---

2. *GLP Consensus Document: The Application of the Principles of GLP to Computerized Systems*, Environment Monograph No. 116 (Environment Directorate, OECD, Paris, 1995), Section 8.

The Retrospective Evaluation Package 87

Figure 5.5. Basic set of SOPs for a legacy system adapted from OECD GLP Consensus: Section 8

Procedures for:

1. Operation of the legacy system (hardware/software), and the responsibilities of personnel involved.

2. Security measures used to detect and prevent unauthorized access and program changes.

3. Authorization for program changes and the recording of changes.

4. Authorization for changes to equipment (hardware/software), including testing before use if appropriate.

5. Periodic testing for correct functioning of the complete system or its component parts and the recording of these tests.

6. Maintenance of the legacy system and any associated equipment.

7. Software development and acceptance testing and the recording of all acceptance testing.

8. Backup of all stored data and contingency plans in the event of a breakdown.

9. Archiving and retrieval of all documents, software, and computer data.

10. Monitoring and auditing of the legacy system.

Figure 5.6. Outline format for a system SOP

Computerized system—standard operating procedure (SOP)

1. Objective—This is guidance for whom to do what?

2. Scope—Inclusions, exclusions, limitations

3. Policy Section

   - regulations to be applied: standards and requirements

   - this SOP is applicable to: roles and responsibilities

4. Procedure Section

   - description of actions to be taken

   - identification of role(s) responsible for each action described

5. Reference Section—List of other SOPs and policies related to this one

6. Appendices—Glossary of specialized terms; templates for reports, logs, and worksheets used in the procedure; system diagrams and flowcharts as needed for understanding the procedure

System SOPs are formal documents signed off by management; they publish the officially accepted way to control system operations. System SOPs are one form of documented evidence for management's control of the system. In practical terms, a general set of SOPs, sometimes called general operating procedures (GOPs), can be developed for the care and use of all the regulated systems in a given area and then only the variations for an individual system's needs are documented in a system-specific SOP.

Writing and approving any missing SOPs is only the first step for management control of a legacy system. The next step is training users and system support personnel on the content of SOPs and having the SOPs themselves available in the work area where they can guide activities during system use. Periodic review and update of the SOPs to reflect changes in the system are further steps frequently checked by auditors.

System Management Logs

The only way to know what actually happens with any system and whether SOPs are really being followed is by recording events and actions as they occur. Such records are usually written in ink in a bound logbook and include the date and signature of the individual making the record. If this has not been done with the legacy system in the past, then a new set of logbook records needs to be established, and people need to be trained in their use.

Two very important logs for any system are the Change Control Log (Figure 5.7) and the Retest Log (Figure 5.8). Change may come to fix a problem, to install an updated version of a system, or to add special enhancements to the system. The size and scope of change determines the amount of testing to be performed before the system can be put back into operational use. Guidelines for this work are found in the Test Plan for the legacy system, which should define what is a major, moderate, or minor change to the system and the level of testing required for each type of change.

Figure 5.7. Change Control Log for System ID: _____

Type of Event: Problem, Fix, Update . . .	Describe the Event So That Any Action Taken Is Clearly Understood	Print Name of Person Reporting This Event	Date	Signature

90   The Survive and Thrive Guide to Computer Validation

Figure 5.8. Retest Record for System ID: _____

Version	Date	Reason for Retest—Periodic Check, Fix, Update . . .	Signature

Other log records to be kept would cover system maintenance, backup of data, backup of system software, system user/security authorization (Figure 5.9), and a general activities log for the *system owner* to record administration and *system team* activities for the system. For all these logs, it is important for individuals who make entries to remember that a log is a record of user experience, actions taken, and events occurring with a computerized system. While a log may include a professional observation as to probable cause or solution to the event reported, a logbook is not a notebook for the recording of one's personal hopes and ambitions for the system. A logbook is expected to be an authenticated record of actual experience with a system.

The system logbook records should be located in a place convenient to the individuals who have to make entries. This is often in the work area where the system is used, but it must be in conditions which keep the entries dry and legible. For major application systems, two separate logbooks may be kept—one for the software application system and one for the platform system. There is no set configuration for logbook records. The goal is to make it as convenient as

The Retrospective Evaluation Package   **91**

Figure 5.9. User Authorization for System ID: _____

Training Experience	Date of Training	Authorized User Name (Printed & Signed)	Security Level	Trainer Sign. & System Owner Sign.

possible for log entries to be written when significant events occur.

System and User Documents

System Documents

User manuals, technical manuals, and system diagrams and flowcharts are often lacking or outdated for legacy systems. In some cases when applications are developed internally, such documents may never have existed in a formal state. The *system owner* and *system team* will need to examine system documents to assess their completeness as well as accuracy for the current state of how the system works.

Replacing documents from external suppliers is relatively straightforward with a purchase order if the supplier is still in business. Having to create manuals that never existed can be very costly and time-consuming. Lack of documentation to explain the system to users and technical support personnel can be one reason for the *system owner* and *system team* to recommend that a *sponsor* retire and replace a system rather than try to validate it for continued use.

User Documents

For legacy systems that lack a User Requirements Document or Needs Analysis Report, it is useful to consider writing a Present-Day Requirements Document based upon the way the system is currently used in the work process. The *system owner* and *system team* can accomplish this by working with a focus group of active users which should also include second- and third-shift personnel. This current-state User Requirements Document can then be used as a benchmark for evaluation testing of the system.

When user manuals are lacking, online help and user notes may be available to use as training materials. These items can be used as a starting point, but they should be expanded by interviewing active users of the legacy system and recording how they work with the system. It is not unusual to find that users have "adapted" a legacy system to perform in unintended and undocumented ways.

All training materials for teaching new users how to operate the system must be checked for their adequacy and their accuracy to the way the system works today. Training records must be reviewed to ensure that today's users of the legacy system have their training experience documented (Figure 5.9).

User SOPs for the legacy system are designed to help people understand how to interact with the system in compliance with validation and quality requirements. Topics to be discussed include security practices, backup and recovery procedures, operation of the system in the work process, and user responsibilities for support, maintenance, and problem resolution as appropriate.

Audit Reports and Quality Control Records

Any retrospective evaluation effort should begin with a baseline audit of the legacy system to establish the size and scope of the effort required to bring it into compliance with company and regulatory validation standards. One logical time to begin this process is when a new version of the legacy system is planned to be installed. After the timeline and history document have been prepared, the Quality Department can perform its baseline audit to good advantage. The *system owner* and *system team* can then use the baseline Audit Report as a goal sheet for the evaluation project.

Deficiencies noted in the Audit Report can be prioritized by the *owner* and *system team* according to what is critical for retrospective work on the current version and what can more logically be put into prospective validation work for the new version of the legacy system. It makes little sense to invest large amounts of time and money to create user manuals and system manuals for the current version if it will be replaced by a new installation in 9–12 months. Such resources would be better spent on documentation for the new version with a minimal effort being applied to the current system. Adequate testing of the current system, however, is not an item to be postponed.

One way to assess the past performance quality of a legacy system is to review the quality control records of the business process using the system. If the computerized process or electronic data handled by the system has consistently met its own QC requirements while using the system, then this can provide a crude but relevant "black box" assessment of the intended functioning of the system. If there have been continuous QC problems with the business process without obvious business reasons for the problems, then there can be serious questions of the quality of the legacy system supporting it. Looking for trends in the QC records can help to identify areas for special testing of the current system. This review of QC data is sometimes referred to as a type of "desk test," meaning that the test is not performed on the system itself, but is an examination of records about the system that one can perform at one's desk, independent of system functions.

Evaluation Testing of a Legacy System

The mechanics of the testing process for a legacy system is the same as for a new system. A written Test Plan is developed and executed with test scripts, normal and problem test data, and Result Logs (Figure 5.10). Finally, a Test Summary Report is written to review all the testing experiences.

If there is no URS to define critical functions of the system, then a new (current) User Requirements Document needs to be created as described above and used as a benchmark for the testing strategy. When there is no formal documentation of past testing experience with the legacy system, the *system owner* and *system team* need to develop a new strategy for what to test, what not to test, and why. When prior testing has been documented, the Retrospective (Retro) Test Plan process is aided by reviewing such documentation and including it in the *evaluation package* and Test Summary Report.

Figure 5.10. Legacy system evaluation testing

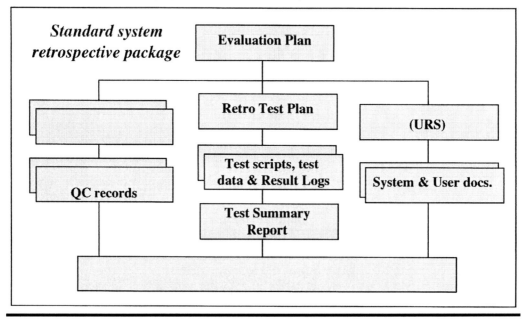

The Retrospective Evaluation Package   95

A Retrospective Test Plan can use much the same outline as a Validation Test Plan, but its approach covers a different view of the life cycle (Figure 5.11).[3] The *system owner* and *system team* have to determine how much installation, operation, and performance qualification (IQ, OQ, PQ) to mix into the current testing package.

Figure 5.11. Retro Test Plan outline (adapted from IEEE Std. 829-1983)

1. Test Plan ID number—Coded to relate to the associated Evaluation Plan

2. Introduction—Items to be tested and reference to related URS

3. Test items—List of software application and system versions to be tested

4. Features to be tested

5. Features not to be tested and why (installed feature not used by application)

6. Approach—Describes overall strategy, techniques, and limits for testing

   - traceability analysis of system functions to URS

   - use of system and user documentation in test scripts

   - risk analysis to define primary focus for testing activities-system impact on safety, efficacy, and quality of strategic business activities, current system versus past and future versions

   - interface testing with systems A, B, and C . . . on the network

7. Item pass/fail criteria—If one test script fails, does whole system fail?

8. Testing suspension criteria and resumption requirements

9. Test deliverables—Documents required: Test Plan, Test Cases, Test Logs, Test Summary Report (templates included in appendices.)

10. Testing tasks—Tasks necessary to prepare for, execute, and report testing

11. Environmental needs—Physical, logical, and security requirements for testing

12. Responsibilities—Identified for test developer, tester and witness

13. Staffing and training needs—Specify skill level for test writer, tester, and witness

14. Schedule—Estimated time to do each task and define milestones

15. Risks and contingencies—Identify high-risk assumptions of Test Plan and specify backup plan to support each

16. Approvals—Specify names and titles of all who must approve this plan, with space for signatures and dates

---

3. IEEE Standard for Software Test Documentation—Std. 829-1983 (The Institute for Electrical and Electronics Engineers, Inc., Piscataway, NJ, 1993), p. 10.

The outline for test scripts and Result Logs of a legacy system are the same as for a new system (refer to Figure 4.7). The Do's and Don'ts of testing remain the same (refer to Figure 4.8) and the Test Summary Report outline is the same (refer to Figure 4.9). The major difference occurs when the legacy system is missing vital system and user documents, system diagrams and flowcharts, or other critical information such as a URS to describe the characteristics of the system and enable them to be understood and properly tested. The creation of this type of documentation then becomes a major preamble to developing test scripts. This may make the whole validation effort too costly to complete.

When a new version of the legacy system is due to be installed in the near future (9 to 12 months), the *system owner* can decide to delay full testing of IQ/OQ/PQ and validation compliance until the new version of the legacy system arrives with its documentation sets. In this case, the *owner* and *system team* can opt to perform the following combination of actions:

- Desk test review of QC records and any past testing records

- Desk test review of System Logs and SOPs for completeness and accuracy

- Desk test review of user documentation for current use and training

- Active scripted testing of current uses for the system using normal and problem data sets

- Writing of a Test Summary Report of the above

Then the *system owner* and *system team* efforts can concentrate on a Transition Plan for retirement of the current version, transition of data and operations to the new version, and a *validation package* for the new version of the legacy system. In this case, the retrospective work on the current system helps to build a stronger foundation for validation of the new version.

Evaluation Summary Report

When all components of the *evaluation package* have been examined and addressed, the *system owner* writes an Evaluation Summary Report (Figure 5.12). The content outline for an Evaluation Summary Report is shown in Figure 5.13.[4] This report tells the *system sponsor* what has been observed and accomplished during the evaluation effort. It should give a concise view of the compliance status of the system with its recommendation in Section 7. There are three possibilities for release status in the Evaluation Summary Report as listed below.

1. This system is released with full validation compliance status.

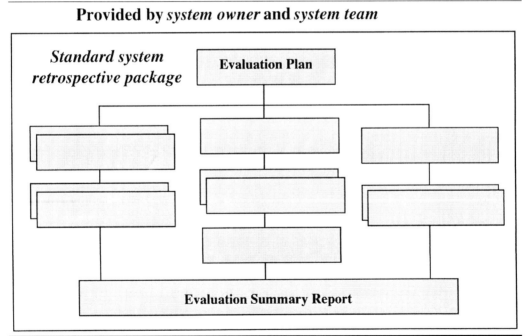

Figure 5.12. Retrospective evaluation package

---

4. IEEE Standard for Software Verification and Validation Plans—Std. 1012-1986 (The Institute for Electrical and Electronics Engineers, Inc., Piscataway, NJ, 1986), p. 18.

98   The Survive and Thrive Guide to Computer Validation

Figure 5.13. Evaluation Summary Report (adapted from IEEE Std. 1012-1986)

1. Plan Identifier: ID number indicating legacy system associated with the Plan

2. Summary of all evaluation tasks

3. Summary of all evaluation package items and their current status

4. Summary of unexpected problems/issues arising and their resolution

5. Summary of deviations from the Evaluation Plan and rationale for deviations

6. Assessment of overall system quality based upon the History Document, Test Summary Report, Audit Report, and System Documentation

7. Recommendations: Release Statement from management for the validation status of the legacy system

8. Approval signature(s) and date(s)

---

2. This system is released with partial validation status which includes the following reservations and conditions: _____.

3. This system is not validated and cannot be used for regulated work environments. It is recommended that this system be retired and replaced.

III. Conclusion

Legacy Systems Need Validation Work to Perform Regulated Tasks Today

The *retrospective evaluation package* begins with a legacy system as it is today and reaches into the past to create a timeline of documented system history to help evaluate its quality and its ability to be validated for continued use. The state of system and user documentation will determine the cost and effort required for a positive outcome. The need for documented control of a legacy system is the same as for a new system if the legacy system is to be continued in service for strategic applications. When the conclusion of the Summary Report is to replace the legacy system, it

The Retrospective Evaluation Package   **99**

gives the *sponsor* a strong body of facts to support future system considerations.

When a legacy system is soon to be updated with a new version, the retrospective effort for the current system can be complementary to the prospective effort for the new version to mutual advantage. For a new version developed within the *sponsor's* company, the deficiencies noted in an evaluation effort can also be communicated to developers for correction in the verification process for the new version so that they do not come up again in the *sponsor's* validation of the new version.

6. The Systems Quality Assurance Plan (SQAP)

I. System Sponsor's Summary

A Logical Approach to Multiple Systems

There are usually more than one computerized system requiring validation in a specific business area, and often there are many of different size, function, and priority. It is important that management has a logical, documented approach to its control of computer validation in regulated areas. Validation resources can easily be consumed by systems where user interest is high or where *owners* see the validation task as easier than for other more complex systems.

There are always more systems to validate than there are resources to do the job, and *system sponsor's* need a rationale for how they prioritize systems and apply resources to validation work. Developing a Systems Quality Assurance Plan (SQAP) to address all the systems in a given area can provide such a rationale and at the same time the SQAP can provide a quality framework which provides consistent structure to all System Validation Plans, packages, and work activities.

The computer validation priorities of external authorities usually come to include the following three concerns which are listed in their order of priority:

1. *Safety*—safety of the system operator or user, safety of the product produced by a controlled process, integrity of data used to prove the safety of regulated product

2. *Efficacy*—consistent potency of product produced by a controlled process, integrity of data used to prove the efficacy of regulated product

3. *Quality*—data and process control having an impact on other quality characteristics of regulated product, such as clarity of sterile solutions or quality of life data

Sponsors using *safety, efficacy,* and *quality* (SEQ) risk analysis as the basis for their system priority in a SQAP will provide a solid foundation for their validation efforts. When a SQAP directs *system teams* to use SEQ risk analysis to organize their system work it also provides a strong focus to all plans for both prospective and retrospective efforts.

II. System Owner and System Team Discussion

The three types of *validation packages* already discussed for prospective verification, validation, and retrospective evaluation work all have a single system as their focus. In practice, most companies in regulated healthcare industries have many strategic systems that operate in regulated environments and require validation efforts. In order to provide a consistent standard of quality to validation efforts, it is necessary for *system sponsors* and *owners* to agree on a strategy for system QA practices. This can be done at several levels within a company through the development of a SQAP to address computerized systems at a particular site, for a specific department or division, or for a large, complex new project, such as the automation of a new manufacturing plant.

SQAPs for Control of a Multiple Systems Environment

As per Figure 6.1, corporate directives and international regulations are translated into a firm's corporate

Figure 6.1. Multiple system environment

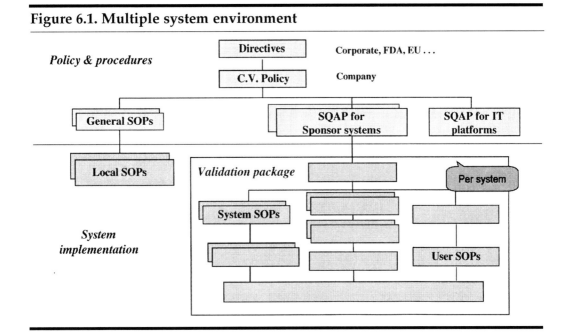

environment by a company's Computer Validation Policy (C.V. Policy).

The C.V. Policy and regulations are then applied to various sponsor environments by SQAPs designed to cover logical groupings of systems. One SQAP for instance might set the standards for how the corporate data center will handle validation for all the platform systems and infrastructure it supplies to the various *sponsor* environments.

One SQAP might address validation practices for all laboratory systems subject to Good Laboratory Practice (GLP) regulations. Another SQAP might look at all clinical development systems and investigator site systems subject to Good Clinical Practice (GCP) inspection. In manufacturing, a SQAP might work for all the Good Manufacturing Practice (GMP)–regulated systems at a plant site. Management might also decide to develop a SQAP for categories of systems used across sites, such as a materials resource planning systems (MRPs), or for bringing a large custom-built project online in a validated state, such as custom-automation for production lines for a new product.

The concept of using the SQAP model is to provide a flexible level of control that gives practical structure and guidance at the *sponsor*, *owner*, and *system team* level for consistent validation practices to meet company policy and external regulatory demands. The goal of any SQAP is to ensure that computer validation is performed according to a standard that is consistent across its scope of authority and will produce *validation packages* that are acceptable to internal audit and external inspection.

SQAP Outline

A SQAP saves time and energy for *sponsors*, *owners*, and *system team*s by defining the validation tasks to be performed within its scope and providing templates for the items expected to be a *validation package*. The SQAP also clarifies roles and responsibilities in the organization for performing validation tasks (Figure 6.2).[1]

Developing a SQAP

The process for developing a SQAP is similar to the process for developing a *validation package*. Depending on the scope of the SQAP, one or more *sponsors* of systems to be covered by the SQAP form a Sponsors' Panel to initiate, guide, review, and approve the SQAP. An area team is then formed of *system owners*, the IT Department, the Quality Department, and key user representatives for major groups affected by the SQAP. This area team then becomes the SQAP Development Team (SQAP Team) (Figure 6.3).

The SQAP Team meets to consider and agree on all the elements contained in the outline shown in Figure 6.2. This process of consensus building can take two days or two months, depending on the level of understanding and experience in the group for computer validation work and the content and existence of a company's C.V. Policy. The

---

1. IEEE Standard for Software Quality Assurance Plans—Std. 730-1989 (The Institute for Electrical and Electronics Engineers, Inc. Piscataway, NJ, 1989), p. 9.

The Systems Quality Assurance Plan (SQAP)   **105**

Figure 6.2. Systems QA Plan (SQAP) (adapted from IEEE Std. 730-1989)

1. Purpose of plan—Business, regulatory, technical

2. Scope of SQAP
   - inclusions—types of systems to be validated
   - exclusions—administrative and nonregulated systems
   - limitations—shared systems controlled elsewhere

3. Reference documents—Regulations, policies, general SOPs

4. Management
   - organization—roles defined for sponsor, owner, team, supplier(s), QC, and QA
   - tasks—validation package activities described
   - responsibilities—role responsibilities identified for package activities

5. Documentation for QC of systems—Logs, plans, reports
   - minimum documentation requirements are defined for standard system packages and special types of systems
   - standard formats and templates are referenced in appendices

6. Standards, practices, and metrics—SOPs for responsible use of validated systems, company policies, and external regulations applied to SQAP scope

7. Reviews, audits, and inspections—type and frequency of system reviews

8. Testing—formal testing practices required for validating systems

9. Problem reporting and corrective action

10. Code and media control—security, archival, and retrieval

11. Supplier control—contracting for quality and service level agreements (SLAs)

12. Records collection, maintenance, and retention

13. Training—Materials and instruction for system users and support personnel

14. Risk management—system and data security, disaster recovery, legacy systems

15. Approvals—Authorized signatures for this Plan

Figure 6.3. SQAP development: people and process

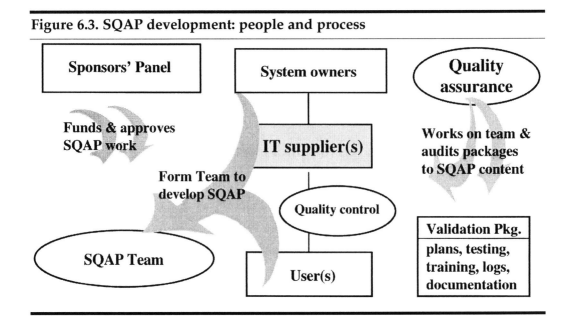

important goal is to reach a consensus, so that *validation packages* are developed to a consistent standard across the domain of the SQAP.

Avoiding "religious" wars about whose format is better for a document's outline can be accomplished by starting with international standards, such as those of the Institute for Electrical and Electronics Engineers, Inc. (IEEE).[2] Although most of the IEEE standards are for software engineering purposes, they easily can be adapted to a systems approach. Such standards reflect a multi-industry consensus of what constitutes good quality practices in information technology.

The good IT practice standards published by IEEE are accompanied by supporting guidelines and documentation to help stimulate thinking on relevant subjects. Since these standards can be applied to space shuttle software as well

---

2. IEEE Standards Collection: Software Engineering (The Institute for Electrical and Electronics Engineers, Inc., Piscataway, NJ, 1994).

as to an automated laboratory instrument, it is important to remember that adapting the standard to fit the size and scope of the task at hand is one of the judgment responsibilities of the *system owners* and others participating on a *system team*. Their scaleability, however, becomes an advantage when the SQAP Team is considering templates for package items.

Purpose

The first section of the SQAP describes to whom the plan applies, such as the Clinical Research Department, all QC laboratories, or production facility XYZ. It also explains why the plan is being written. There are usually three dimensions to the reason for why a SQAP is developed. The first, *business*, has to do with the company's business dependency on computerized operations, and the need to have reliable systems and protected data of good quality to keep its working processes running smoothly and profitably.

The second purpose, *regulatory*, is concerned with the organization's compliance to some specific authority or governmental regulations for computer validation which are required for the company to sell its product and remain in business. The third aspect, *technical*, is one of management control over technology in order to have reliable systems available to users with the least interruption of workflow, so that the organization shows a positive return on its investment in technology.

Scope

In this second section of the SQAP, the Team has an opportunity to define the limits of the SQAP effort. No organization has the time and resources to do fully documented *validation packages* on every system in its operation. Here is where exclusions and limitations can be described and the reason for their classification recorded. An auditor or inspector may not always agree with every point in the

108   The Survive and Thrive Guide to Computer Validation

exclusion and limitations description, but he or she will respect an organization that has recorded its practice and followed it in implementation.

Inclusions

All systems put into the category of inclusions are subject to the full extent of the SQAP good practices. The SQAP Team needs to consider the different types of computerized systems used in the area covered by the SQAP and describe a way for *sponsors* and *owners* to identify those systems that require a computer validation effort. In addition, there should be a guideline for determining a reasonable priority scheme for planning the validation work. The example in Figure 6.4 illustrates these points in language that is generic and can be adapted to different Team situations.

Figure 6.4. SQAP Scope: Example of Inclusions

This SQAP applies in full to computerized systems

1. that control a regulated process and have a direct impact on the safety, efficacy, or quality of regulated product;

2. that handle data used to prove to authorities the safety, efficacy, or quality of regulated product; and

3. whose failure would result in a safety concern for any personnel.

Given that time and resources are limited, system validation work shall be prioritized according to a standard schema. Validation priority is given in the order below when system failures have a direct impact on the

1. Safety—of personnel, of product, and of product data in that order;

2. Efficacy—of product potency or strength and of data about product efficacy to be used for discussions with authorities; and

3. Quality—other quality aspects of the product in production and of data about other quality attributes of the product to be used for discussion with authorities.

Note: This SEQ schema is to be applied at gross system level and then to function and activity levels throughout the validation effort for systems included in this Systems Quality Assurance Plan.

The Systems Quality Assurance Plan (SQAP)   109

Exclusions

Although the quality assurance practices of a SQAP can be applied to such strategic systems as payroll, regulatory authorities usually are not interested in employee benefit package systems and business convenience. This makes administrative systems a logical category to place under exclusions. Other usual exclusions are the internals of commercial software used in platform systems, such as operating systems, network protocols, and spreadsheet and database systems.

Limitations

Sometimes an area uses a system hosted at a corporate location outside the control of the SQAP Team. For such shared systems, the SQAP would apply only to modifications implemented within the SQAP area, such as individual spreadsheets developed for regulated purposes or database modifications made to an MRP package for local, regulated applications.

Reference Documents

The reference section of the SQAP lists all documents referenced by the Plan. It would include any government regulations that apply, any corporate or local policies that apply, and any general operating procedures (GOPs) or SOPs that are related to the SQAP content. Any IEEE, ISO, or other standards used or adapted for the SQAP and its package templates should also be listed. It is important to use the qualifier "adaptations from" to clarify when a standard has been used as a guide rather than as a strict standard, but the use of recognized standards as a foundation for SQAP work is an inspector-friendly effort.

Management

The management section provides a template for action, and it is the part that always takes the longest to develop. It is the most critical one and sometimes the most difficult one for which to build a consensus. The management section defines who is whom in validation by role and not by name or title. It describes the tasks involved in developing a *validation package,* and it assigns responsibility for specific tasks to specific roles. If an individual is *sponsor* of one system, *owner* of a second system, and user representative of a third, he or she should be able to read this section of the SQAP and know exactly which tasks to perform for the role assigned to each system—*sponsor, owner,* user.

Organization

This subsection lists the roles required to perform computer validation under the SQAP. It also identifies the characteristics of each role by its relationship to a computerized system, so that people reading the document know which role they fit into for any system.

- *System sponsor*—management person with the regulatory responsibility for the data handled, or the process controlled by a computerized system

- *System owner*—individual appointed by the *sponsor* to ensure the daily availability of a computerized system for its intended purpose

- *System supplier(s)*—individuals providing platform systems, software, or services to a computerized system

- *System user*—person operating a system for its intended purpose in the business process

- *System quality control*—quality professional actively involved in the validation effort and ongoing monitoring and testing of system quality

- *Quality assurance*—quality professional not associated with development of a system's validation package who audits the system and its package for compliance to regulations, company policy, and SQAP requirements

- *System Team*—reports to *system sponsor,* is lead by *system owner,* and includes all other roles above, with the exception of quality assurance

The Systems Quality Assurance Plan (SQAP)   **111**

- *SQAP Team*—reports to Sponsor Panel and includes multiple *system owner*s, QA, system users and suppliers as needed.

- *Sponsor Panel*—*System sponsor*s sharing a common area of computer validation interest

Tasks and Responsibilities

Initially, the SQAP Team compiles a list of each step required to prepare a *validation package*, including necessary approvals. Then a role is assigned responsibility for each task. It is often helpful to combine tasks and responsibilities into a table for the final SQAP document. The table provides a template for *system teams* to use later or adapt to their situation without wasting a lot of time recreating the basic process. Table 6.1 gives a 20-step example of the system validation process as it might appear in a SQAP.

Documentation

The documentation section of the SQAP defines what the minimum documentation requirements are for various types of *validation packages* (SDLC verification, prospective validation, and retrospective evaluation). It also can define optional or special documentation for specific types of systems, such as very small software applications. Very small applications could be individual spreadsheets or macros for statistical software, drivers for instruments, or ladder logic for programmable logic controllers (PLCs) used for regulated purposes. For very small systems, the elements of a Validation Plan can be condensed into a brief form, such as the example in Figure 6.5.

Standards, Practices, and Metrics

The standards, practices, and metrics section provides guidance to *system team*s across the scope of the SQAP by establishing standards for contract wording for validation requirements for external vendors and service agreements

112   The Survive and Thrive Guide to Computer Validation

Table 6.1. SQAP Table of System Validation Tasks and Responsibilities

Validation Task	Role Responsible
1. Identify system sponsor, assign system owner, and form a system team.	System sponsor and system owner
2. Develop and write a Validation Plan.	System team
3. Review and approve the Validation Plan.	System sponsor and QA
4. Develop and write a Test Plan.	System team
5. Approve the Test Plan.	System owner and system QC
6. Develop user and tester training program and training materials.	System owner supported by system team and supplier
7. Deliver training to users and testers.	System owner supported by system team QA and supplier as appropriate
8. Develop system and user SOPs and system logbook records.	System owner and system team
9. Review and approve system and user SOPs.	System sponsor and QA
10. Develop test scripts, test data, and Result Logs.	System team
11. Review and approve test scripts.	System owner and system QC
12. Prepare testing environment. Assign and train witnesses.	System owner and system QC
13. Execute test scripts, record results, and witness.	Trained user testers and witnesses
14. Review test results and write a Test Summary Report.	System team and system owner
15. Review and approve the Test Summary Report.	System sponsor and system QC
16. Conduct vendor audit of system supplier and write Audit Report.	QA
17. Conduct self-inspection program of ongoing system audits and write reports.	QA
18. Compile standard validation package and review all evidence of tasks.	System owner and system team
19. Write Validation Summary Report.	System owner
20. Review and approve the Validation Summary Report.	System sponsor and QA

The Systems Quality Assurance Plan (SQAP)   113

Figure 6.5. Very small systems (VSS) validation form outline

Name of Program: _____

1. Author of this program is: *(signature and date)*
2. Program was developed using: *(language or application with version number)*
3. System owner of this program is: *(signature and date)*
4. Program performs the following function(s): *(list and describe functions)*
5. Program interacts with the following system(s): *(system name; type of interaction)*
6. User instructions for this program include the following: *(procedure for normal use; problem and help process)*
7. Program has been tested for normal and problem cases by: *(signature and date)*
8. Testing activity and Result Log were witnessed by: *(signature and date)*
9. Program released for validated use by owner: *(signature and Date)*
10. Change control record: *(log for fixes, updates and retesting)*

with internal suppliers of regulated systems. One way to accomplish this is by developing or referring to general operating procedures (GOPs) that apply across all departments and systems related to the SQAP. Topics for GOPs could include the following:

- Supplier management and contract wording for validation requirements
- Document management for System Logs and *validation packages*
- Basic set of SOPs for software applications and platform systems
- Project management and development standards for systems to be validated
- Testing standards and practices for validating systems
- Ongoing auditing, monitoring, and inspection practices for validated systems

Reviews, Audits, and Inspections

The review, audit, and inspection section describes the technical and managerial reviews and audits to be performed for validated systems throughout their life cycles. If appropriate GOPs or SOPs already exist to cover this topic, then this section references them. Otherwise, it discusses reviews and audits of internal and external system suppliers, as in the example below.

> System teams shall determine the extent of ongoing management review and audit activities to be performed per system when writing the Validation Plan and preparing a system's validation package.
>
> 1. For off-the-shelf, nonconfigurable applications purchased from external suppliers: No vendor audit is required. The OTS software will be subject to QA audit as part of the review of the validation package.
>
> 2. For configurable applications from an external supplier: No vendor audit is required, but one may be performed at the discretion of the system team. The configured component of the system will be subject to QA audit as part of the review of the validation package.
>
> 3. For custom-built, regulated systems from internal or external suppliers: Full QA review and audit throughout development and deployment of the system is required.

A GOP for common system auditing practices would include the following conditions:

- Auditors must be independent of the system activity being audited.
- Audits shall be conducted to known industry standards and/or company SOPs.
- An Audit Report shall be written for all audits performed.

The Systems Quality Assurance Plan (SQAP)   115

- Audit Reports are shared with *system owner* and *system sponsor*, and remain company confidential to all parties.

- *System owner* is responsible for follow-up work to correct deficiencies cited in the Audit Report.

- An audit follow-up review is conducted and reported to assess corrective actions taken.

- An Audit Log is kept per system to record date of audit or follow-up review, name of auditor, and name of *system owner* as witness to the audit activity.

- An Audit Log is kept to acknowledge that follow-up work to an Audit Report has been completed with *system owner's* signature and date

For regulated systems, it is good to have the *system team* identify a subset of the group to serve as an Inspection Response Team and be prepared to present and defend the system's *validation package* during inspections. An SOP should be available to define roles and responsibilities for how to handle a system's inspection by external authorities.

System Testing

The testing section of a SQAP describes the different types of testing performed on computerized systems and discusses where such testing would be used for regulated systems in its domain. There are three types of testing usually applied to software application systems:

1. *White box or structural testing*—Testing that takes into account the internal mechanism of a system or component. Types include branch testing, path testing, statement testing (IEEE).

2. *Black box or functional testing*—Testing that ignores the internal mechanism of a system or component and focuses solely on the outputs generated in response to selected inputs and execution condition (IEEE).

3. *Gray box or combination testing*—A mix of functional and structural testing.

116 The Survive and Thrive Guide to Computer Validation

White box testing should always be performed extensively by the system developer during the Build and Test Phases of the SDLC. Structural testing may be performed on a more limited scale during system acceptance testing in the Commission Phase of the system's life cycle as decided by the *system team*. Black box testing is performed to some degree by system developers to assure meeting user requirements, but it is extensively performed during performance qualification in the user environment.

During the commissioning of a new GMP-regulated manufacturing system, both the software application and its hardware platform system are challenged with testing. The primary focus for testing varies across three levels of qualification that have been adopted with increasing frequency by *system teams* working outside of manufacturing areas.

1. *Installation Qualification (IQ):* Documented verification that all key aspects of the installation adhere to approved design intentions according to system specifications, and that manufacturer's recommendations are suitably considered.

2. *Operational Qualification (OQ):* Documented verification that each unit or subunit operates as intended throughout its anticipated operating range.

3. *Performance Qualification (OQ):* Documented verification that the integrated system performs as intended in its normal operating environment.

In Figure 6.6, an example is given for the testing section of a SQAP developed for the manufacturing area subject to GMP inspections.

Problem Reporting and Corrective Action

The problem reporting/corrective action section of the SQAP describes the accepted approach to providing a system for processing user and system problems that have an impact on SEQ functions. Usually, a Configuration Management Logbook is established by the *system owner* to record all system problems and their resolutions. Depending on the size and complexity of the system, a user Help

Figure 6.6. SQAP for GMP computerized systems: Testing section

As per this SQAP, both structural and functional testing need to be performed for all systems. The location of the testing and combination thereof depends on the source of code development and/or system design.

- Nonconfigurable systems from external suppliers (instrument automation) require black box testing by the system team.

- Configurable systems from external suppliers (LIMS, individual spreadsheet or specific macro program) require gray box testing by the system team.

- Custom-built systems (process control systems) require white box testing by the supplier and black box testing by the system team.

- Internally supplied systems require both white box and black box testing by developers and the system team.

During the commissioning of a new GMP system, both the software application and its hardware platform system are to be challenged with testing according to the following schema:

For GMP application software:

- Software IQ tests check the physical installation and logical configuration for compliance to the supplier's specification for platform software required by the version of software being installed.

- Software OQ tests check intended execution for boundary conditions and other parameters per functional module and for the integrated system.

- Software PQ tests check performance of the software to intended operation in normal and stress conditions of the working environment.

For GMP hardware and platform systems:

- Hardware IQ testing checks for compliance of the physical installation to the documented manufacturer's specification for power, environmental conditions, static control, calibration, and system description in associated documentation.

- Hardware OQ testing checks that hardware components, configured as a unit, perform platform functions in support of OQ testing for the hosted GMP software application.

- Hardware PQ testing checks that the configured platform supports the PQ testing of the hosted GMP software application.

Under this SQAP, the Validation Plan and/or Test Plan for a specific GMP system will define the level of white/black/gray box testing to be used per IQ/OQ/PQ phase. The Test Plan for a specific system will define the detailed strategy for testing, and test scripts will describe the specific procedures for such testing. Testers will record their observations on a Result Log, and witnesses will check test records for completeness. Testing practices SOP XXXX will be followed.

Desk may be established as first line of support for user issues, and only those issues resulting in communication with the supplier or adjustments to the system configuration would be noted in the logbook.

This section should require *system teams* to define on a per system basis what would be classified as major, moderate, or minor system problems. In general, classifications would include the following:

- *Major Problem*—system malfunction resulting in loss or corruption of data, or failure of the system to perform its intended function

- *Moderate Problem*—system malfunction resulting in work interruption due to a specific screen function not being available, failure of reports to print, or network downtime for integrated systems

- *Minor Problem*—system action resulting in altered screen layout, different screen sequence, or other malfunction that has no SEQ impact

The corresponding level of corrective action per degree of problem should also be defined. Since it is important not to create parallel operations, the SQAP should connect its problem handling process to whatever quality control procedures an organization has established for handling problems (Figure 6.7).

Code and Media Control

The code and media control section addresses the issue of access to custom-built code if a system's supplier should go out of business. Contracting for an escrow bank vault–type of storage for a master copy of any purchased code can provide the purchaser with some assurance of being able to retrieve the code for maintenance and repair purposes should the supplier's organization dissolve. System code developed internally should be just as protected with a master copy that is archived and kept current with updates and new versions.

The Systems Quality Assurance Plan (SQAP)   119

Figure 6.6. SQAP example: Corrective action levels

The company's deviation reporting system (SOP XXXXX) is to be used for processing system problems which impact SEQ processes. In general, reporting and response classifications shall include:

For *major problems* with the system:

- Reporting: File a deviation report and log the system problem in the system Configuration Management (C.M.) Logbook

- Corrective action: Exercise system recovery SOP and retest the system as per the Test Plan in its *validation package*. Note corrective action in C.M. Logbook

For *moderate problems:*

- Reporting: File a report with the system Help Desk resource and log the problem in the system's C.M. Logbook

- Corrective action: Exercise problem resolution process as per system Validation Plan and retest system as per Test Plan in the *validation package*. Note corrective action in system's C.M. Logbook.

For *minor problems:*

- Reporting: Note problem in system's C.M. Logbook

- Corrective action: Fix problem and note corrective action in C.M. Logbook

---

The system's Validation Plan should specify the methods and facilities to be used to

- identify and manage safe storage and retrieval of media (tapes, diskettes, or CDs) used for the software application, platform components, and data files in the database, and

- protect the media from unauthorized access, unintended damage, or physical degradation.

Such controls should be documented in a system SOP for backup, recovery, and disaster recovery.

120 The Survive and Thrive Guide to Computer Validation

Supplier Control

The supplier control section references vendor audits and the escrow account process. It also references a GOP or SOP about supplier management practices, if one is available. Otherwise, it describes items to be included in vendor contracts and internal and external service level agreements. It would require that all requests for proposal (RFPs) to suppliers of custom-built systems clearly state what regulations and standards apply for the validation of a system under the directives of the SQAP.

This section also defines *sponsor, owner,* and user responsibilities in support of supplier activities for life cycle tasks associated with planning, purchase, and acceptance of a new computerized system. The Needs Analysis Report and User Requirements Specification are two important inputs that enable a supplier to produce a reasonable System Design Description and allows acceptance criteria to be established. The International Organization for Standardization (ISO) has published a Standard ISO 9000-3 that gives a framework for software supplier contracts that can be included here or referenced in a supplier management GOP (Figure 6.8).[3]

Records Collection, Maintenance, and Retention

For the records management section of the SQAP, a GOP or local SOP for managing validation documentation can be referenced for more detail. During the Operational Phase of the life cycle for critical systems, validation package documentation should be maintained in a secure, controlled location designated by the *system team.* Data records and system copies should be managed as per the system backup and recovery SOP. Prior to the installation of a new version of a system, a Transition Plan is developed to address the archival needs for system data, media, and documentation.

---

3. Quality Management and Quality Assurance Standards—Part 3: Guidelines for the Application of ISO 9001 to the Development, Supply and Maintenance of Software, ISO 9000-3:1991(E) (International Organization for Standardization, Geneva, 1991), p. 4.

The Systems Quality Assurance Plan (SQAP)   121

Figure 6.8. ISO 9000-3 Standard for quality items in contracts

Contract items on quality are given in section 5.2.2 and include the following:

a. Acceptance criteria

b. Handling of the changes in purchaser's requirements during the development

c. Handling of problems detected after acceptance, including quality-related claims and purchaser complaints

d. Activities carried out by the purchaser, especially the purchaser's role in requirements specification, installation and acceptance

e. Facilities, tools, and software items to be provided by the purchaser

f. Standards and procedures to be used

g. Replication requirements:

- The number of copies of each software item to be delivered

- The type of media for each software item, including format and version, in human-readable form

- The stipulation of required documentation, such as manuals and user guides

- Copyright and licensing concerns addressed and agreed to

- Custody of master and backup copies where applicable, including Disaster Recovery Plans

- The period of obligation of the supplier to supply copies

Training

In its training section, a SQAP establishes the standard that a system's Validation Plan is expected to define the training requirements for system users and support personnel. Training records are to be kept to document the identity of trainees and the content of training received. Training and user materials are to be developed and used in training prior to system operation for SEQ purposes. The training component is an integrated part of a system's *validation package* under the Validation Plan and should be included in the Validation Summary Report.

122 The Survive and Thrive Guide to Computer Validation

Risk Management

The risk management section of a SQAP discusses the types of risks most likely to occur in a system's working environment. It then discusses preventive measures to be taken to prevent or address the system risks mentioned. Table 6.2 illustrates the kind of items to be considered.

Approvals

The SQAP is just a paper document until it is reviewed, approved, and signed off for release and implementation. While it is important not to have too long of a signature list, there should be at least one signature from the three organizational components involved in the development of the SQAP process. The example below illustrates this signature philosophy.

Table 6.2. Validation Risks and SQAP Preventive Actions

Validation Risk	SQAP Preventive Action
Loss of data or system	Backup, recovery, and disaster recovery SOPs
Hardware/software change— major, moderate, minor	Change control SOP, Configuration Management Logbook, and change classification with retest criteria in Validation Plan and/or Test Plan
Environmental conditions	Tested in OQ/PQ and conditions monitored
Unauthorized access to systems and/or SEQ data	Physical and logical access control devices as needed and security SOP for password control and user profile authorization
Inspection by external authorities	Standard validation package and assigned Inspection Response Team to answer queries on the package

The Systems Quality Assurance Plan (SQAP)   **123**

This SQAP is approved for implementation at the XYZ organization.

Signs for Sponsors' Panel:

Signature: _____ Date: _____

Signs for Quality Assurance Department:

Signature: _____ Date: _____

Signs for SQAP Development Team:

Signature: _____ Date: _____

Appendices

The appendices of a SQAP can contain as many different kinds of items as are useful to support the plan. Some common elements would be the following:

- Descriptions of standard system *validation packages* and templates for the items they contain
- A business plan for how to implement the SQAP in the organization over the next fiscal year
- A glossary of terms and acronyms used in the SQAP and in computer validation work
- The list of resources available to support *system teams*

III. Conclusion

A SQAP Focuses System Team Efforts to Save Time and Prioritize Systems

Developing a SQAP across multiple system groups allows an organization to reach a consensus on validation practices. It prevents wasted recycling of multiple team efforts to reinvent the process and lets the organization's energy and resources focus on getting systems validated. Validated systems perform reliably and maintain the integrity of strategic SEQ data and automated SEQ processes. Finally, validated systems are compliant with required regulations.

A good SQAP document demystifies the computer validation process for an organization and gives a framework for system quality that is practical to implement. The consistent practice of validation work across the organization gives an audit-friendly and inspection-friendly impression and provides documented evidence for management's control of strategic systems. It also becomes the benchmark by which system quality can be measured and the quality return on system investment can be observed.

7. Computer Validation Policy

I. System Sponsor's Summary

Policy—The Role for Senior Management in Computer Validation

Senior management in organizations subject to Good Practice regulations for computer validation have a significant role to play in support of systems compliance. In fact, senior management has the overall responsibility for systems compliance and thus for ensuring that computerized systems are suitable to their intended purpose. Management executes its role through a combination of policy and commitment, where "commitment" is defined as providing an adequate number of appropriately qualified and trained staff and ensuring an adequate standard in facilities, equipment, and data handling procedures.

The most detailed regulatory statement about management's responsibilities was published in Paris in 1995 by the Organization for Economic Cooperation and Development (OECD) in its Good Laboratory Practice (GLP) Consensus Document on The Application of GLP Principles to Computerized Systems.[1] The OECD group included the regulatory views of Europe, the United States, and Japan and its concepts of management responsibility for computer policy, procedures, and compliance are shown in Figure 7.1.

---

1. *GLP Consensus Document: The Application of the Principles of GLP to Computerized Systems,* Environment Monograph No. 116, (Environment Directorate, OECD, Paris, 1995), p. 14.

Figure 7.1. OECD GLP Consensus: computerized systems

Management is responsible for

- Establishing computing policies and procedures to ensure systems are developed, validated, operated, and maintained to GLP standards
- Ensuring policies and procedures are understood and followed
- Ensuring effective monitoring of compliance to requirements of policies and procedures

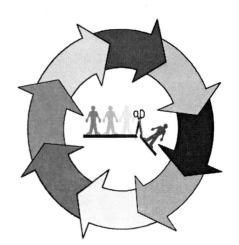

These statements for GLP can also be applied to Good Clinical, Manufacturing, and Electronic Submission Practices. The term *GXP* is used in policy and procedure work as a convenient way to express all the Good Practice regulations with a single acronym, where the "X" represents L, C, M, or any other regulation for Good Practice. Validation practices for computerized systems are usually the same across all GXP areas, and management's role remains consistent as well. The short list of management's responsibilities is shown in Figure 7.2.

A corporate Computer Validation (C.V.) Policy sets policy and procedures in a way that translates the meaning of compliance to regulatory directives into the culture of the organization. Policy brings sanity to the process of computer validation in the organization as a whole, just as a systems quality assurance plan (SQAP) brings a standard approach and consistent level of quality to validation in a defined area of the organization. A policy reduces wasted organization cycles by providing a framework for general operating procedures (GOPs) and standard SQAP practices across the whole organization.

Figure 7.2. OECD GLP Consensus: computerized systems

Management is responsible for

- Setting policy and procedures
- Compliance to regulations
- Supply and training of staff
- Providing suitable facilities
- Planning for disaster recovery

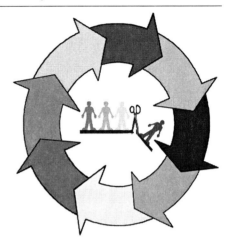

A policy from senior management gives legitimacy to system validation efforts and brings them into the mainstream of business decision-making and project budgeting priorities. It requires *system sponsors* to plan ahead for staffing, training, facilities, and disaster recovery of strategic systems and gives them an approved strategy for doing so.

Information technology expenditures have grown to major proportions today for most organizations, and senior managers have raised concerns about how to understand the return on such investment. Through the implementation of a C. V. Policy, *system sponsors* can give senior management a view of the return on investment for strategic systems. This view will be in the form of documented evidence for systems reliability, data integrity, and successful audits and inspections.

II. System Owner and System Team Discussion

The work of *system owners* and *system teams* is much easier to accomplish when it is performed within a framework of clearly defined policy and procedures. It is also easier to accomplish when time, budget, and people for validation have been planned and scheduled as a normal part of the system life cycle and business process workflow.

The challenge for any organization is to translate regulatory and corporate directives into a reality-based policy that is practical to implement within the culture of the organization. It is too easy to write the perfect policy that gets filed away and never looked at again because it does not reflect the way people in the organization agree to operate. Such a perfect policy would leave management open to inspection trauma based upon lack of "due diligence" to implement.

Developing a Computer Validation Policy

It is important that the policy development initiative come from the most senior level of management who will review and approve its final form. Experience has shown, however, that it is equally important for the content of C.V. Policy to be developed by a representative group of *system sponsors, owners,* and *system team* members who understand the reality of validation work and have to agree to follow the policy directives (Figure 7.3).

A Validation Executive Committee (VEC) is formed of six to eight of the most senior managers of the organization and chaired by the chief executive. This group is made up of senior managers for all areas in the organization using regulated systems plus the senior managers for Quality and Information Technology (IT). In the drug and biopharmaceutical industries, a VEC would include the vice presidents of Research, Clinical Development, Manufacturing, Regulatory Submissions, Quality, and IT.

The VEC initiates the policy project by defining the overall business purposes of the organization for writing a policy on computer validation. Then it appoints two of its members to form and lead a working group (Policy Team) to develop the content for the policy. Usually, the senior

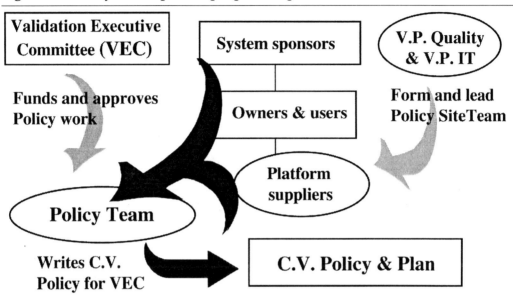

Figure 7.3. Policy development: people and process

managers for Quality and IT are a logical choice for heading the Policy Team.

Members of the Policy Team should be drawn from among *system sponsors, owners,* users, and platform suppliers representing each area of the VEC membership. In fact, VEC members should be chartered to help select the most experienced and capable people in their area for participation on the Policy Team. In this way, they ensure that their needs are addressed by the Policy, and they communicate to their people the importance of the effort and of implementing the Policy once it is developed and approved. In most major drug firms, this will produce a Policy Team of 25–30 people.

The Policy Team develops a consensus for how applicable regulations and directives translate into the organization's operations. It then develops a common glossary of terms and definitions for validation work and models for compliance activities that can be fit into the reality of normal

130   The Survive and Thrive Guide to Computer Validation

business constraints and the given corporate culture. Finally, the Policy Team develops a Way Forward Business Plan for how to implement the Policy once it is approved. The VEC then reviews and approves the Policy and resources the Implementation Business Plan.

Content for a Computer Validation Policy

Experience has shown that corporate culture will dictate the look and feel of a policy document, but there are some common issues which need to be addressed by any C.V. Policy. The questions below raise these common issues whose answers form the content of a C.V. Policy document. The questions have been arranged into the four major sections of a policy document where their answers would be placed.

1. Executive message—Signed by Validation Executive Committee

    - What is the purpose or rationale for writing the C.V. Policy?

    - What is management's commitment to implementation of the Policy?

    - What is the responsibility of line management for GXP systems validation?

    - What are management's business objectives for GXP systems and services?

2. Policy introduction

    - What is the scope (inclusions, exclusions and limits) of GXP systems and services to be covered by the Policy?

    - How does one define a GXP system or service for the purposes of the Policy?

    - What are the Policy's business objectives for GXP systems and services? (management control, data integrity, system reliability, auditable quality)

Computer Validation Policy   **131**

3. Policy requirements

- What is the **life cycle model** used by the Policy for GXP Systems and how is it to be addressed by computer validation practices?

- What is the Policy's **system team model** for validation practices at the individual system level?

- What is the **management model** above system level which supports system validation work and implementation of the Policy?

- What is the **documentation model** for validation work?

- What is the approach to **standard system packages** for verification, prospective validation, and retrospective evaluation of GXP systems?

- How is the validated status of a GXP system to be maintained over time?

- What are the roles for quality professionals in system validation, audits, and inspections? (SQC and QA)

- What is the **inspection response model** at the system level?

- How are internal and external suppliers of GXP systems and services to be managed for computer validation concerns?

- How is this Policy to be implemented, monitored for compliance, and updated over time? (process defined)

4. Appendices

- What are the accepted terms and definitions for validation work under this Policy? (glossary)

- Are there any associated GOPs or SOPs to help implement this Policy? (list)

- What are the templates to be used for essential validation documents shown in the documentation model and standard system packages? (outline formats)

132   The Survive and Thrive Guide to Computer Validation

- How is this Policy to be implemented, monitored for compliance, and updated over time? (Implementation Business Plan and Monitoring Reports)

When the VEC and Policy Team consider their answers for business and technical objectives for GXP systems, it is good to keep in mind the four major themes of all computer validation regulations. They are shown in the GXP validation matrix in Figure 7.4. In fact, GOP and SOP titles can be arranged on this matrix as a training aid for rolling out Policy implementation. The matrix provides a visual tool for keeping in mind the main concerns of regulators and business management.

Policy Requirements Models

There are essentially six models of requirements that need to be developed for an organization in order to clarify the way that validation practices will be implemented under

Figure 7.4. Computer Validation Policy: GXP validation matrix

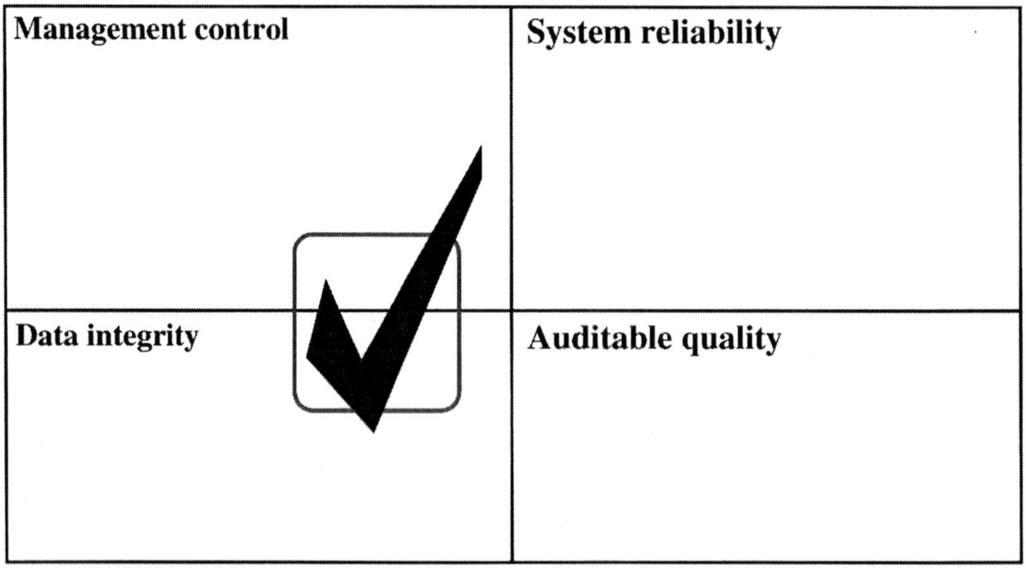

Management control	System reliability
Data integrity	Auditable quality

Computer Validation Policy   **133**

the Policy (Figure 7.5). Developing a picture for each of these models will help all Policy Team members understand computer validation expectations and how to implement them. The models then become useful training aids for helping others in the organization understand how to work in compliance with the C.V. Policy.

System Life Cycle Model

Chapter 2 of this book discusses in detail the phases of a system life cycle based upon the life cycle described in the European Union (EU) GMP Guide Annex 11 for Computerized Systems (Figure 7.6).[2] There are other ways to picture and discuss system life cycles, and a Policy Team is free to describe a model in any way that is suitable for its local culture.

The importance of a life cycle model is its ability to show the scope of validation activities across all phases of system acquisition, system development, and system use through to retirement. The usefulness of the model in Figure 7.6 is that it also illustrates the life cycle phases where the system supplier the *system owner* differ in their areas of direct responsibility.

Figure 7.5. C.V. Policy models for validation requirements

1. System life cycle model

2. System Team model

3. Management model

4. Documentation model

5. Standard system packages

6. Inspection response model

---

2. *Guide to Good Manufacturing Practice for Medicinal Products—Annex 11: Computerized Systems, The Rules Governing Medicinal Products in the European Union Volume IV* (Office for Official Publications of the European Communities, Luxemburg, January 1992), pp. 139–142.

Figure 7.6. System life cycle model

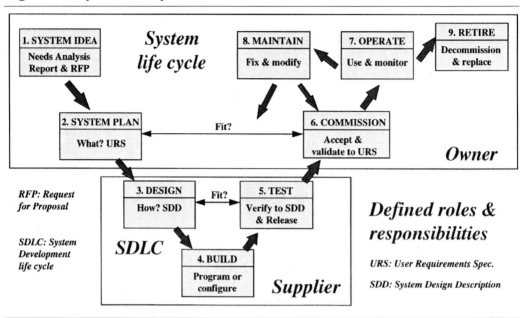

System Team Model

Chapter 1 of this book introduces the organization of *system sponsor*, *owner*, and *system team* as a model for validation work at the system level (Figure 7.7). This model is also the one described in words in Chapter 6 as the organization for system level work performed under the control of the SQAP. The model was also adapted a bit to describe the development team for an SQAP.

A Policy Team can also adapt this model to meet its own needs. The key attribute of the model is that role names are used instead of specific job titles or personal names. This allows the Policy Team to define validation roles and responsibilities in a generic way, which is protected from organizational change and turnover in personnel. It also helps the person who may have different roles for different systems understand what functions to perform in various team efforts—*sponsor*, *owner*, user, supplier, SQC, or QA.

Figure 7.7. System team model

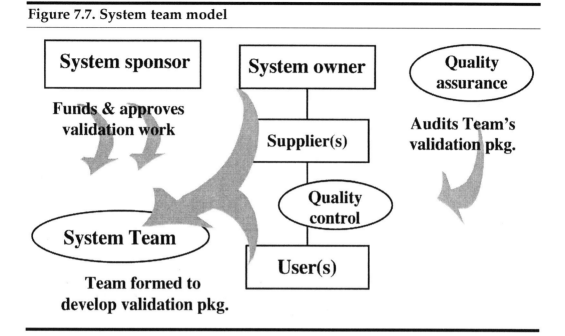

Management Model

System Teams need the support of a management framework such as SQAP groups that recognize and plan for validation efforts to be included with the mainstream of other work responsibilities in the area. Computer validation for strategic systems is too important and demanding an effort to be hidden and conducted in a spare time, nonbudgeted manner. After the Policy Team develops the C.V. Policy, and it is approved by the VEC, the various SQAP groups translate the Policy into their own areas with a new or updated SQAP and implement it with their *system teams* (Figure 7.8).

As no policy is perfect in the first version, the SQAP Groups will find issues arising as they work to implement the C.V. Policy. The Policy Team continues to operate and provide an issue resolution role as well as a compliance monitoring role. On a periodic basis the Policy Team prepares a Compliance Report for review by the VEC. The

136 The Survive and Thrive Guide to Computer Validation

Figure 7.8. Management model

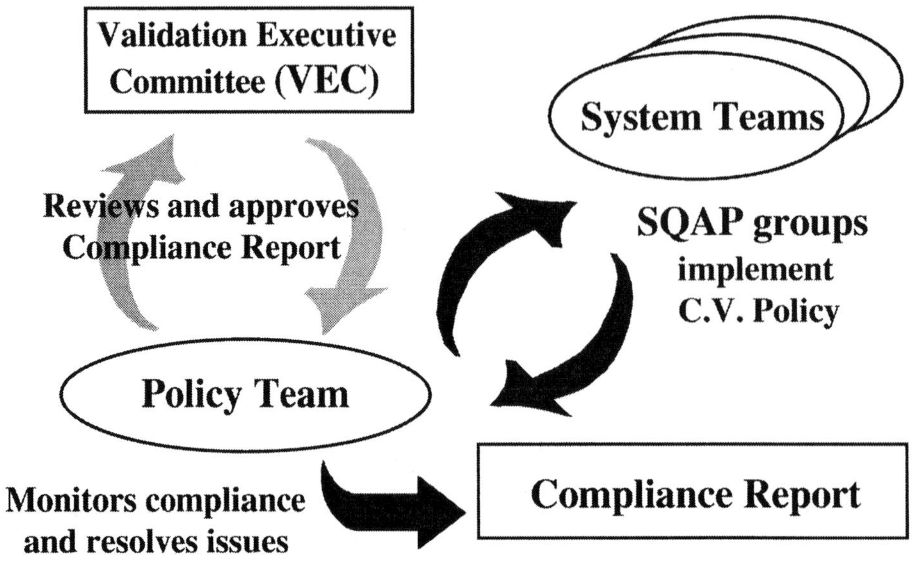

Validation Executive Committee (VEC)

Reviews and approves Compliance Report

Policy Team

System Teams

SQAP groups implement C.V. Policy

Monitors compliance and resolves issues

Compliance Report

Policy Team sets the timing of the report as needed, usually on an annual basis. Interim reports can always be developed for crisis situations that should have the attention of the VEC, such as major inspection activities.

Sometimes issues arise among SQAP groups for such things as system jurisdiction and allocation of scarce technical resources, the Policy Team can be used as an arbitration forum. If the Policy Team is unable to resolve the concerns, then the VEC becomes the final decision maker. Since it is not pleasant to bring problems to senior management, this model usually allows enough opportunity for problem resolution to occur below the VEC.

Here again, a Policy Team can take the model in Figure 7.8 and massage it to fit the local culture. The key issue is that a management structure is in place to support validation work as a normal part of business and has within it the opportunity to resolve territorial and budgeting disputes.

Computer Validation Policy

Documentation Model

The C.V. Policy cannot float in mid-air by itself in an organization without a plan for the rest of validation documentation. The whole thrust of C.V. Policy implementation is providing documented evidence of system quality; this must be done in an orderly fashion if it is to pass audit and inspection. One structured approach to validation documentation that ties it all together is shown in Figure 7.9.

Corporate and external directives are translated into the organization as a whole by the C.V. Policy, which is sponsored and approved by the VEC. Significant areas within the organization then form SQAP groups and translate the C.V. Policy into the needs of their specific domains with SQAPs as described in Chapter 6. General SOPs help to reduce redundancy of effort and keep consistent standards for implementation across SQAP groups.

Under an SQAP there is system implementation of computer validation with local SOPs and standard *validation*

Figure 7.9. Documentation model

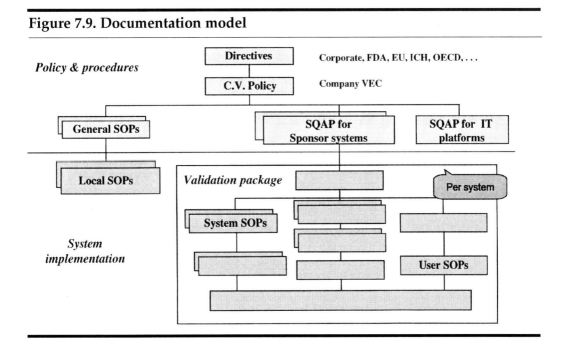

packages developed for individual strategic systems. Within the standard *validation package*, there are SOPs for system management and SOPs for user operation of the system.

The documentation model identifies all the important types of documents coming under a C.V. Policy and shows their relationship to each other. A structured approach at the C.V. Policy level makes it easier to organize documentation at lower levels and helps people understand how their efforts fit into the whole.

One of the GOPs or local SOPs should address the management of standard *validation packages* so that storage, protection, and availability of package items are handled properly for both operational and inspection purposes. At Policy or GOP level, document templates should be described for all items in the Standard *validation packages*.

Standard System Validation Packages

Chapter 3 of this book discusses in detail a standard package for supplier verification of systems during their development cycle, and Chapter 5 covers the standard package for a retrospective evaluation of legacy systems. Chapter 4 defines the standard package for prospective validation of a new strategic system and describes each of the items in the package (Figure 7.10).

Consistent structure and format for package items across SQAP systems are important for ease of use and of audit. *System team*s should not have to waste energy recreating ways to develop a package or package items. Standard outlines should be provided for the Validation Plan, Test Plan and other documents. These may have to be adapted to some specific situations for individual systems, but there should be a consistent starting point for every prospective Validation Plan, Test Plan, and testing documentation. In like manner, there should be a consistent outline starting point for the Verification Plan, Test Plan, and testing documentation. The same is true for the *retrospective package*.

Figure 7.10. Standard validation package

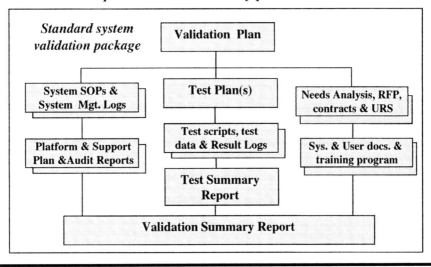

Inspection Response Model

For pharmaceutical and healthcare industries, audits and inspections of strategic computerized systems should never come as a surprise to the organization. The C.V. Policy must provide an action model to address system inspections in a responsible way. When inspectors come to the door, there should be an orderly procedure for them to be met and their visit hosted by a QA professional (Figure 7.11).

Since the documented evidence of a system's quality is contained in the standard system *validation package*, the *system owner* should be prepared to present the package to the inspector or auditor in an organized manner. At the time of package preparation, the *system team* should designate an Inspection Response Team from among its members to be ready and available to answer queries on package items that they helped to prepare.

The *system sponsor* receives the Inspection Report and refers it to the *system owner* for follow-up action. For inspections

Figure 7.11. Inspection response model

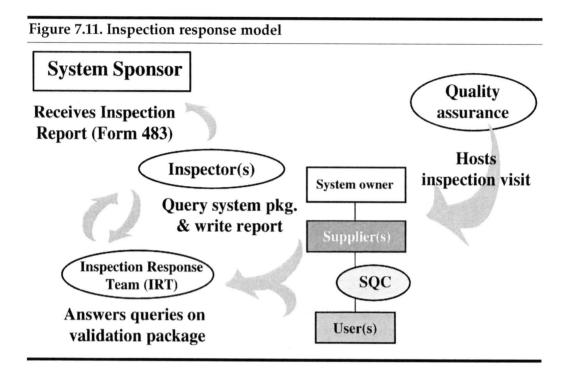

performed by the U.S. Food and Drug Administration (FDA), both positive and negative observations made during an inspection are reported in a document format called a Form 483. The items on a Form 483 can become objects of extreme interest to the VEC if they are preliminary to a plant shutdown or product recall due to systems noncompliance.

III. Conclusion

Implementing a C.V. Policy Brings Good Business Benefits

Organizations must be able to trust the systems that can affect product quality and be able to prove that such systems are reliable. They must be able to trust their data and be able to prove that their data handling systems are reliable.

The best way to accomplish these business needs is through the development and implementation of a C.V. Policy for strategic systems.

Regulatory directives hold senior management responsible for the quality of strategic GXP systems. It is possible for senior management to fulfill its "due diligence" role for control of regulated systems by sponsoring the development and implementation of C.V. Policy. Additional business benefits are obtained when the Policy is developed to reflect the local culture of the organization. Integrating validation work into the normal business workflow for strategic systems brings budget and resource planning into the light for a more successful result.

The business benefits that come with the standardized approach of a good C.V. Policy include

- reliable systems and reliable data for strategic operations,

- reduced cycle times for validation work due to standard procedures and document formats,

- first time pass of inspections and audits, and

- positive return on systems investment measured in auditable quality.

8. International Regulations and Directives

I. System Sponsor's Summary

Regulatory Timeline

Regulations for computer validation began with the U.S. Food and Drug Administration (FDA) in February 1983, when it published a document for its inspectors entitled *Guide to Inspection of Computerized Systems in Drug Processing*.[1] This guide became known by the color of its cover—the "Blue Book"—and continues to be used by inspectors today. At that time, computer-controlled processes had become noticeable in pharmaceutical manufacturing to the point where systems reliability was becoming a significant factor in the quality of the regulated product.

Since 1983, the influence of computerized systems in all phases of drug research, clinical development, and product manufacture has increased dramatically, as illustrated by the impact circles of Figure 8.1. In fact, many drug firms today produce diagnostic and therapy delivery systems that include microchip and other computerized elements as part of their product. Since 1991, the international regulations and directives for validation of computerized systems have increased 300 percent. Some of the most useful of these recent regulations are shown in the regulatory timeline in Figure 8.1.

---

1. *Guide to Inspection of Computerized Systems in Drug Processing* (Blue Book) (U.S. Government Printing Office, Washington, DC, 1983-381-166:2001, February 1983), pp. 1–25.

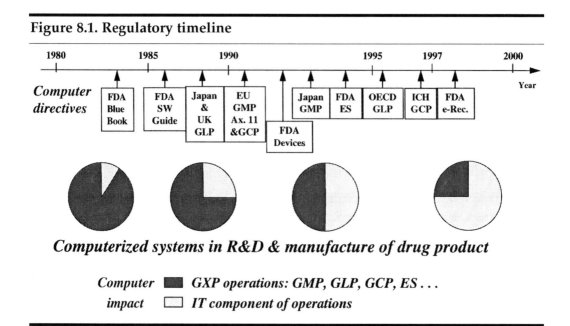

Figure 8.1. Regulatory timeline

System sponsors and owners participating on a Policy Team should be aware of these directives and use them to good advantage in developing their implementation concepts for computer validation in their organization's C.V. Policy as per Chapter 7. Full copies or extracts of the relevant parts of these directives are included in Chapters 13–15 of this book for easy reference.

FDA regulations are official documents that have the force of law and the courts behind them. The FDA electronic records document 21 CFR Part 11 and the FDA GMP for computerized medical devices are regulations that are enforceable by legal action of the U.S. government. Firms can have market access denied, manufacturing plants closed, or product recalled through legal action of the FDA following inspections showing serious infractions of its computer validation regulations.

Official directives are regulatory documents that give strong guidance, but are not necessarily enforced by law. The ICH GCP and OECD GLP are both official directives

International Regulations and Directives   145

that may be adopted by local countries for legal enforcement but are not themselves subject to legal action. In 1997, both the European Union (EU) and the United States adopted the ICH GCP as part of their respective regulatory requirements for clinical trials, and many countries have added the OECD GLP Consensus concepts to their already existing GLP regulations.

For *sponsors* and *owners*, it makes sense to build a computer validation strategy based upon the foundation of agreed standards for good practice that have already been recognized and accepted by international authorities. This ensures that the approach is understood and agreeable to inspectors from the start, and any controversy over concepts is avoided.

II. System Owner and System Team Discussion

EU GMP Guide Annex 11: Computerized Systems

The easiest computer validation document for *owners, system teams* and general managers to read and understand is the EU GMP Guide Annex 11 on Computerized Systems.[2] It is barely four pages long, and in 19 paragraphs, it covers all the important elements of validation work using nontechnical language. Included in Chapter 13 of this book, Annex 11 can be incorporated into any training program to explain the needs of GXP computer validation work quickly, regardless of the lab, clinical, manufacturing, or submission discipline of the participants.

Figure 8.2 shows how Annex 11 maps onto the validation matrix (Figure 7.4) introduced in the policy development discussion of Chapter 7. The requirements of Annex 11 have been categorized under the four major themes of all computer validation regulations. The numbers in parentheses correspond to the paragraph numbers in Annex 11,

---

2. "Guide to Good Manufacturing Practice for Medicinal Products—Annex 11: Computerized Systems," *The Rules Governing Medicinal Products in the European Union Volume IV* (Office for Official Publications of the European Communities, Luxemburg, January 1992), pp. 139–142.

146 The Survive and Thrive Guide to Computer Validation

Figure 8.2. EU GMP Annex 11 requirements

Management control	System reliability
• Principle—product quality	• Software quality assurance (5)
• Personnel (1)	• Testing (7)
• Validation/life cycle management (2)	• Control of change (11)
• System environment (3)	• Alternative arrangements (15)
• Supplier contracts (18)	• Recovery procedures (16)
• Release security (19)	
Data integrity	**Auditable quality**
• Built-in entry & processing checks (6)	• System description (4)
• System security (8)	• Audit trail—entry & edits (10)
• Verification of critical data (9)	• Paper copies—data audits (12)
• Data integrity (13)	• Error tracking (17)
• Data backup (14)	

and the titles next to the parentheses summarize the content of the paragraph referenced by the numbers.

The official focus for Annex 11 statements is the prospective and ongoing validation of computerized systems used for data handling and process control subject to GMP regulations across member states of the European Union (EU). On careful reading, one quickly sees that the same statements can be made for computerized systems operating in other types of regulated areas as well and that they could be located elsewhere in the world.

The quality concepts for technology discussed in Annex 11 are universal for computerized systems everywhere. The life cycle discussed in Paragraph 2 is a standard one for software technology and has been the basis for the discussions in Chapter 2. Paragraph 19, which discusses security for automated batch release of product under GMP, can easily translate to "database locking" of study data under GCP and automated release of Certificates of Analysis or laboratory testing reports under GLPs.

OECD GLP Consensus: Application of GLP Principles to Computerized Systems

The OECD Consensus Document was published in Paris in April 1995, and reflects a common vision of GLP validation concepts across major world authorities—the European Agency for the Evaluation of Medicinal Products (EMEA), the FDA, and Japan's Ministry of Health and Welfare (MHW).[3] It is a much longer document than Annex 11, and includes the added knowledge of inspection experience gained during the years since January 1992 when Annex 11 became effective. In its 13 pages, the OECD Consensus includes all of the same concepts as Annex 11, but it gives more detailed coverage of each concept and adds several more items to the list of quality requirements as per Figure 8.3.

Where Annex 11 states *what* to do for computer validation, the OECD document usually provides *system* and *policy teams* with more detailed guidance for *how* to meet various validation requirements. This can be seen especially in the section about minimum documentation that includes a list of topics for 10 basic system SOPs (refer to Figure 4.11).

The growing use of networked systems and integrated applications in the 1990s is reflected in the OECD's introduction of the item related to communications between computers or between computers and peripheral equipment. It states that

> all communication links are potential sources of error and may result in the loss or corruption of data. Appropriate controls for security and system integrity must be adequately addressed . . .[4]

The concept of retrospective evaluation for legacy systems is found in the OECD Consensus and not covered in Annex 11. This reflects the practical experience of finding systems where the need for GXP compliance was not foreseen or

---

3. *GLP Consensus Document: The Application of the Principles of GLP to Computerized Systems*, Environment Monograph No. 116 (Environment Directorate, OECD, Paris, 1995), pp. 3–15.

4. OECD, Section 3(b)(ii).

148   The Survive and Thrive Guide to Computer Validation

Figure 8.3. OECD GLP: extras beyond Annex 11

Management control	**System reliability**
• Management responsibilities (1a, b) • Validation support mechanism (7d) • Management policies (8a) • Source code availability (8c)	• Communications (3b) • Retrospective evaluation (7b) • Basic 10 system SOPs (8d)
Data credibility	**Auditable quality**
• Raw data definition (5) • E-data archives (9)	• QA responsibilities (1d) • Training records (2)

not specified. In such cases, an assessment of system suitability must be made based upon historical records and a plan developed for ensuring the future validation of the system.

An issue of rising importance in this decade is the storage and retrieval of electronic data (e-data), and the OECD Consensus was the first official document to address this area in any detail. In Section 9 on archives, it states that electronic GLP data must be stored with the same levels of access control, indexing, and expedient retrieval as other types of GLP data. Among other points, it says that

> No electronically stored data should be destroyed without management authorization and relevant documentation. Other data held in support of computerized systems, such as source code and development, validation, operation, maintenance and monitoring records, should be held for at least as long as study records associated with these systems.[5]

---

5. OECD, Section 9.

International Regulations and Directives   **149**

FDA—Electronic Records; Electronic Signatures; Final Rule

The FDA has a regulation effective as of August 20, 1997, that provides the criteria under which the FDA

> will consider electronic records to be equivalent to paper records and electronic signatures equivalent to traditional handwritten signatures.[6]

This long-awaited official ruling reflects the increased use of automated systems in place of paper-based processes for regulated applications. It is an inclusive regulation that applies to records in electronic form that are created, modified, maintained, archived, retrieved, or transmitted, under any FDA regulations and not only GLP, GCP, GMP, or electronic submission (ES).

Computer systems (including hardware and software), controls, and associated documentation used under this regulation are expected to be readily available for and subject to FDA inspection. This regulation also addresses security over a network and defines two types of system networks—one that is internal to the organization (closed), and one that allows access from outside the organization (open). These and other FDA definitions in the regulation are given below.[7]

- **Biometrics** means a method of verifying an individual's identity based on measurement of the individual's physical feature(s) or repeatable action(s) where those features and/or actions are both unique to that individual and measurable.

- **Closed system** means an environment in which access is controlled by persons who are responsible for the content of electronic records that are on the system.

---

6. 21CFR Part 11-Electronic Records; Electronic Signatures; Final Rule. *Federal Register* Thursday, March 20, 1997, p. 13430.

7. 21 CFR 11, p. 13465.

150   The Survive and Thrive Guide to Computer Validation

- **Digital signature** means an electronic signature based upon cryptographic methods of originator authentication, computed by using a set of rules and a set of parameters such that the identity of the signer and the integrity of the data can be verified.

- **Electronic record** means any combination of text, graphics, audio, pictorial, or other information representation in digital form that is created, modified, maintained, archived, retrieved, or distributed by a computer system.

- **Electronic signature** means a computer data compilation of any symbol or series of symbols executed, adopted, or authorized by an individual to be the legally binding equivalent of the individual's handwritten signature.

- **Handwritten signature** means the scripted name or legal mark of an individual handwritten by that individual and executed or adopted with the present intention to authenticate a writing in a permanent form. The act of signing with a writing or marking instrument such as a pen or stylus is preserved. The scripted name or legal mark, while conventionally applied to paper, may also be applied to other devices that capture the name or mark.

- **Open system** means an environment in which system access is not controlled by persons who are responsible for the content of electronic records that are on the system.

The FDA's electronic record regulation has in it all of the computer validation concepts of the EU Annex 11 and the OECD GLP written in very brief language and adds to it some new ideas around the security and control of electronic records and electronic signatures, as shown in Figure 8.4.

While EU Annex 11 establishes the basics of system validation, and the OECD Consensus adds detail and clarifies

International Regulations and Directives   151

Figure 8.4. FDA e-record: extras to Annex 11 and OECD

Management control	**System reliability**
• Controls for closed systems (11.10)	• Device checking (11.300e)
• Controls for open systems (11.30)	• Authority checks (11.10g)
• Electronic signatures (11.100)	• Signature/record linking (11.70)
	• E-signature components & controls (11.200)
Data credibility	**Auditable quality**
• Electronic records (Subpart B)	• Signature manifestations (11.50)
• Independent time-stamped audit trail of entries and actions (11.10e)	• Identification codes & password controls (11.300)

roles and responsibilities for management and others in computer validation, this FDA regulation looks at the replacement of paper with computer technology and seeks to ensure the following:

- The e-record is accurate and available for review during the full regulatory retention period for the record type.

- E-signatures are fully binding on and undeniable by their *owners*.

- E-records and e-signatures are securely linked together so that changes cannot be made to falsify records and approvals.

- E-records and e-signatures are secure and protected from unauthorized access, use, or modification.

The regulation states that system documentation must show that an individual understands and agrees to the fact that the use of his or her e-signature carries the same mean-

152   The Survive and Thrive Guide to Computer Validation

ing as a handwritten signature and binds the individual to the consequences of such a signature. When an e-signature is not based on biometrics, such as voice print or retinal scan, it must use at least two distinct identification components, such as a password and an identification code.

If a person is absent and his or her e-signature must be executed, the regulation requires that at least two other individuals having appropriate authority must combine their respective e-signature capabilities in order to execute the single absentee e-signature. This would result in two alternate passwords and two identification codes being used to execute the absentee's e-signature privileges.

FDA's Blue Book for cGMP Systems

While all the other countries of the world use the term *GMP* for their manufacturing regulations, the U.S. FDA uses the term *cGMP* for *current* Good Manufacturing Practices with the idea that practice standards change over time as skills improve. For simplicity's sake, all future references in this book will include the FDA's *cGMP* in the generic term *GMP* as one common global acronym.

Back in 1983 when the first of the FDA's computer regulations came out, systems were not as complex as today, and networks were not as sophisticated. The extent of system use in the manufacturing process was limited but growing fast, and the FDA felt it had to give its inspectors guidance on how to review computerized production. While the Blue Book does not give a neat list of system SOPs as in the OECD Consensus, it does note throughout its text specific topics that should have written procedures for inspectors to review. These topics are shown in Figure 8.5 and can be seen to cover many familiar ideas later included in the EU GMP Annex 11.

The Blue Book has a strong focus on stand-alone systems and control devices. Its concerns for computerized operations include manual backup systems, input/output checks, process documentation, monitoring of computerized operations, alarms, shutdown recovery, and networks.

International Regulations and Directives   153

Figure 8.5. U.S. FDA Blue Book: Topics for SOPs

1. Definition of the operational limits for critical systems

2. Defined process for accepting hardware and software systems

3. Documented testing practices

4. Maintenance procedures for hardware and software systems

5. Revalidation procedures for ongoing conditions and change situations

6. Security practices for protecting system programs and data

7. Performance of system overrides and manual overrides for computer-controlled processes

8. Documented change control mechanism for changes in equipment, software, and the exercise of manual or system initiated process control overrides

9. Backup operations for systems and data records

10. Alarm response procedures for correcting production problems

11. Manual production operations to be followed in case of system shutdown

12. Recovery from unplanned system shutdown

It also tells inspectors that they should spot-check a firm's monitoring practices for automation to include the following six computerized items:[8]

1. Calculations—for verification by an alternate method

2. Input recording—for sensor readings versus computer indications

3. Component quarantine control—for actual warehouse location versus batch data record

4. Timekeeping—for clock accuracy in real time control

5. Automated cleaning-in-place—for assuring adequacy of cleaning and elimination of residue

6. Tailings accountability—for what limits, if any, the firm places on residual material (tailings) carried over between batches in continuous processing

---

8. Blue Book, p. 14.

154   The Survive and Thrive Guide to Computer Validation

Figure 8.6. Inspector questions for hardware systems—Blue Book

1. Does the capacity of the hardware match its assigned function?

2. Have operational limits been identified and considered in establishing production procedures?

3. Have test conditions simulated "worst case" production conditions?

4. Have hardware tests been repeated enough times to assure a reasonable measure of reproducibility and consistency?

5. Has the validation program been thoroughly documented?

6. Are systems in place to initiate revalidation when significant changes are made?

Figure 8.7. Inspector questions for software systems—Blue Book

1. Does the program match the assigned operational function?

2. Have test conditions simulated "worst case" production limits?

3. Have tests been repeated enough times to assure consistent reliable results?

4. Has the software validation been thoroughly documented?

5. Are systems in place to initiate revalidation when program changes are made?

The Blue Book also provides inspectors with a list of suggested questions to ask about hardware and software. These are shown in Figure 8.6[9] and Figure 8.7.[10]

FDA Computerized Medical Device GMP

By the early 1990s, the sophistication of medical device technology had reached a point where the FDA issued a special Medical Device GMP Guidance for FDA Investigators titled *Application of the Medical Device GMPs to Computerized Devices and Manufacturing Processes.*[11] This document can be useful to *system owners* and *system teams* for its

---

9. Blue Book, p. 6.

10. Blue Book, p. 11.

11. *Medical Device Good Manufacturing Practices Manual*, 5th ed. (U.S. Government Printing Office, Washington, DC, ISBN 0-16-035844-2, FDA 91-4179, August 1991), Appendix pp. 1–24.

International Regulations and Directives   155

discussion of how GMP regulations apply to computers and the types of controls that would typically be expected for automated processes and internally developed systems.

It discusses five important items for environmental control of computer hardware, which are temperature, humidity, electrostatic discharge (ESD), dust and dirt control, and electromagnetic interference (EMI). It also defines the meaning of "worst case" for any type of validation testing.[12]

> **Worst Case:** A set of conditions encompassing upper and lower processing limits and circumstances, including those within standard operating procedures, which pose the greatest chance of process or product failure when compared to ideal conditions. Such conditions do not necessarily induce product or process failure.

The Device GMP gives a specific description of the calibration procedure for computers in an automated manufacturing process that can help *system owners* and *system teams* understand regulatory views and apply them to their own situation (Figure 8.8).[13]

It also discusses the process of protecting a master copy of original software and closely managing production copies of it to ensure that production copies are not altered during their use. This practice can be applied to GXP spreadsheets and PLC software in any FDA–regulated process.

Advice for the calibration of computer hardware is given by the Device GMP Guideline as shown in Figure 8.9.[14]

Japan's Ministry of Health and Welfare (MHW)— GMP Guideline

Japan's MHW set April 1993 as the enforcement date for its *Guideline on Control of Computerized Systems in Drug*

---

12. Device GMP, p. 22.

13. Device GMP, p. 12.

14. Device GMP, p. 8.

Figure 8.8. Medical Device GMP: computerized process validation

When a manufacturing process is automated, the computerized system is validated to assure it performs as intended. In validating computerized equipment, parameters that the system is designed to measure, record, and/or control are evaluated by an independent method, until it is demonstrated that the computer system will function properly in its intended environment.

When a manufacturing process is controlled by computer, functional evaluation of the control system may include, but is not limited to, the following activities:

- equipment (peripherals, etc.) and sensor checks using known inputs, which may consist of processing test or simulated data;

- alarm checks at, within, and beyond their operational limits; and,

- evaluation of operator override mechanisms for how they are used by operators and how they are documented.

In case of system failure, evaluations would include:

- how data is updated when in manual operation;

- what happens to data "in process" when the system shuts down;

- what procedures are in place to handle shutdown; and,

- how product or information handled by the computerized process is affected.

Figure 8.9. Calibration of computer hardware—Device GMP

Calibration of computer hardware is similar to calibration of any other electromechanical system.

1. The sensor's measurement of temperature, voltage, resistance, etc., is compared against the measurement of a known standard traceable to the National Institute of Standards and Technology or other acceptable standard.

2. An important part of the calibration activity is to assure that measurements are properly transmitted across computer communication lines and properly interpreted by the computer system.

3. Verification of properly transmitted measurements is accomplished by comparing the measured value that has been input into the computer system with the value of the traceable standard.

International Regulations and Directives   157

Manufacturing.[15] Its objective is to provide guidance for development and use of custom-built systems in process control, production control, and quality control under drug GMP and other regulations.

Guideline Scope

The scope of this Guideline is unusual in that it states exclusions as well as inclusions. Authorities rarely exclude items from their review process. Figure 8.10 shows the system inclusions and exclusions for Japan's GMP Guideline. The guideline applies to systems used in drug manufacturing plants subject to Japan's Drug GMP regulations.

SDLC Documentation

A major emphasis of the MHW directive is the development process for custom-built systems. In Part 3, it describes roles and responsibilities for system design and engineering, program development, and system

---

Figure 8.10. System scope of MHW GMP Guideline

Includes:

- Systems for manufacturing process control and management including recording batch data

- Systems for production control such as storage and inventory of starting materials, intermediates, and final products

- Systems for documentation of manufacturing directions, testing protocols or records

- Systems for quality control and recording of QC data

Excludes:

- Systems with limited function which are operated simply by input of parameters to a fixed program provided by the supplier of hardware as general functions of the devices

---

15. "Guideline on Control of Computerized Systems in Drug Manufacturing," *Manual for Control of Computerized System in GMP* (Yakuji Nippo-sha, Tokyo, 1993, ISBN 4-8408-0278-5), pp. 23–32.

158   The Survive and Thrive Guide to Computer Validation

performance testing and gives guidance for documented control of the development process. Figure 8.11 describes the documentation prescribed by the Guideline for system development life cycle (SDLC) activities.

Installation and Operation Guidance

The MHW Guideline discusses installation and operation testing. All testing is to be performed according to written

---

Figure 8.11. MHW GMP Guideline: SDLC documentation

1. *System Development Manual*—with engineering standards, documentation standards, design change control procedures, exit criteria for each phase of the development process

2. *Development Schedule*—with development objectives, time schedule, staffing resources, selection criteria and equipment plan for hardware

3. *System Engineering Document*—with hardware composition, outline of system functions, tabulation of input/output data, file structure outline, countermeasures against system shutdown, security control functions, and title or name of the manager and person(s) in charge. (This document to be prepared in compliance with the System Development Manual.)

4. *Program Specification*—with details of input/output data, data processing, and title or name of manager and person(s) in charge. (This document to be prepared in compliance with the System Development Manual.)

5. *Trial Test Plan for the Program*—with test methods, a provision for test records, and evaluation criteria of test results. The manager shall evaluate results of the trial test and thereafter approve it.

6. *System Performance Test Plan*—to confirm the system performance in compliance with its design specifications in nonproduction conditions. This plan includes testing conditions, check items and test data to be used, test methods, test records, problem logs, evaluation criteria for results, testing schedule, and assignment of tasks during testing. The manager evaluates and approves results according to following criteria:

    a. *Function*—does it match provisions in the system engineering document?

    b. *Capability*—assurance of system response as designed in the system engineering document

    c. *Reliability*—does the recovery function work properly?

    d. *Operation*—appropriate operation of terminal devices, etc.

International Regulations and Directives   159

Test Plans and procedures with test data and testing records retained. The manager approves the system after evaluating the test results.

Part 4 of the Guideline focuses on controlling the operation of GMP systems. This includes operating procedures, change control, inspection and maintenance, the handling of accidents, security control and self-inspection practices. Figure 8.12 shows some of the topics suggested for SOPs.

Document Storage and Retention Times

Part 5 of the MHW GMP Guideline addresses the storage and handling of system documents and records that may be on paper or electronic media. Documents and records relevant to system development are to be retained for three years from the date of retirement of the system from operation (or for one year after the expiration date of a drug made using the system). Records relevant to system operation are to be retained for three years from the date of recording (or for one year after the expiration date of a drug made using the system).

ICH Good Clinical Practice (GCP) Directive

The International Conference on Harmonization (ICH) developed a consensus document for GCP that was accepted by both the European Union and the U.S. FDA in 1997 as binding on all clinical studies conducted in their respective countries. Japan's MHW also participated in the ICH effort and approved the consensus document.

Section 5.5.3 of the ICH GCP addresses the validation of electronic data handling during clinical studies for drug development (Figure 8.13).[16] Like many other regulations in the mid-to-late 1990's it requires computer validation to be implemented, but gives few details for how the implementation is to be accomplished. It is up to *system owners*

---

16. ICH Topic E6—Guideline for Good Clinical Practice (The European Agency for the Evaluation of Medicinal Products, Human Medicines Evaluation Unit, Available on the Internet from http://www.EUDRA.org/EMEA.html), p. 24.

160 The Survive and Thrive Guide to Computer Validation

Figure 8.12. MHW GMP Guideline: SOP topics

1. Operation of hardware and software to SOPs

2. Education and training of personnel

3. Daily inspection and periodic maintenance of hardware and software
   - maintenance of the environment
   - inspections before and after operation
   - inspection of input data

4. Accident prevention, alarms, and accident recovery measures
   - alarm setting of the system
   - system halt conditions and organization in case of accidents
   - procedures for recovery, cause finding studies, and future prevention
   - evaluation of product impact from system accidents
   - procedures for necessary manual backup systems
   - training for backup manual systems

5. Security control for both physical and logical access to systems and data
   - control of passwords and identification codes
   - assigned privileges to enter, modify or delete data
   - limited access to hardware
   - backup copies of programs and data

6. Change control for system alterations and testing of system after change
   - approval of change and execution of change
   - review and test of system after change is made
   - update to system documentation for changes made
   - notification of changes to persons concerned

7. Self-inspection and monitoring records

International Regulations and Directives 161

Figure 8.13. ICH Guideline for GCP: Section 5.5.3

When using electronic trial data handling and/or remote electronic trial data systems, the sponsor should:

a. Ensure and document that the electronic data processing system(s) conforms to the sponsor's established requirements for completeness, accuracy, reliability, and consistent intended performance (i.e., validation).

b. Maintain SOPs for using these systems.

c. Ensure that the systems are designed to permit data changes in such a way that the data changes are documented and that there is no deletion of entered data (i.e., maintain an audit trail, data trail, edit trail).

d. Maintain a security system that prevents unauthorized access to the data.

e. Maintain a list of the individuals who are authorized to make data changes (see 4.1.5 and 4.9.3).

f. Maintain adequate backup of the data.

g. Safeguard the blinding, if any (e.g., maintain the blinding during data entry and processing).

and *system teams* to develop their own approach to validation work for meeting the regulatory requirements.

ICH Guideline on Statistical Principles for Clinical Trials

In Section 3.6 of the ICH Draft Guideline on Statistical Principles for Clinical Trials, it states that the ICH GCP Section 5 should be applied to the process of data capture through database finalization:

> Specifically, timely and reliable processes for recording data and rectifying errors and omissions are necessary to ensure delivery of a quality database and the achievement of the trial objectives through the implementation of the analysis plan.

162   The Survive and Thrive Guide to Computer Validation

This concern is carried on further in Section 5.8 as quoted below:[17]

> **5.8 Integrity of Data Capture and Computer Software:** The credibility of the numerical results of the analysis depends on the quality and validity of the methods and software used both for data management (data entry, storage, verification, correction, and retrieval) and for processing the data statistically. Data management activities should therefore be based on thorough and effective SOPs. The computer software used for data management and statistical analysis should be reliable, and documentation of appropriate software testing procedures should be available.

III. Conclusion

World Authorities Are Increasing C.V. Directives for GXP Systems

Although the first computer validation directive came out in 1983, since 1991 validation regulations and directives from international authorities have increased dramatically and continue to develop. An examination of a range of international regulations and directives gives a picture of some consistent concepts and useful directions for systems validation work. The four themes of management control, data integrity, system reliability, and auditable quality prevailed across all items examined:

- EU GMP Guide Annex 11—a good management and training overview of validation concepts for systems in operation

- OECD GLP Consensus—more detail for responsibilities and activities

- U.S. FDA e-records; e-signatures—controls for using new technologies

---

17. *International Conference on Harmonization; Draft Guideline on Statistical Principles for Clinical Trials* (Available on the Internet from http://www.fda.gov).

International Regulations and Directives 163

- U.S. FDA Blue Book—basic concepts for inspector reviews

- U.S. FDA Device GMP—inspectors view of controls for internal production and use of systems as products

- Japan's MHW GMP—focus on software development and operation of customized systems

- ICH GCP—includes computer validation as a partner with other GCP requirements

- ICH Statistical Principles for Clinical Trials—discusses system validation as essential to valid analysis

Policy Teams need to take the best input from regulations and directives such as these and translate them into a practical approach for their organizations. Then *system owners* and *system teams* can use the C.V. Policy's approach to validate their GXP systems in a consistent and realistic way across all parts of the organization.

9. Survive and Thrive with Reviews, Audits, and Inspections

I. System Sponsor's Summary

Audit Perspectives and ROI—What They See Is What You've Got

Reviews, audits, and inspections provide the weeding and pruning exercises necessary to keep GXP computerized systems surviving validation with vigor and a GXP work process thriving on the resulting quality of system reliability and data integrity. What a reviewer, an auditor, or an inspector sees during his or her time with a system provides the *system sponsor* with an independent view of what has been received as return on investment (ROI) for the system. The basic concern of all inspections is simply stated by the EU GMP Guide Annex 11 shown in Figure 9.1.

Perfection is not the criteria for GXP systems inspections, but at the very least, computers should not make matters worse. For most system sponsors investing in strategic GXP systems, this is not enough, and they expect a return on computerization that provides an improvement over prior ways of operating.

Three types of external checking activities can help *system sponsors* and *owners* to objectively gauge the quality and GXP compliance of a system. These include reviews by management or other professionals in the same organization, a formal audit by the QA function external to the

165

Figure 9.1. What's the basic concern?

EU GMP Guide Annex 11: Computerized Systems

Principle:

Product quality and quality assurance should not decrease when a computerized system replaces a manual operation.

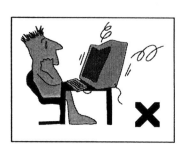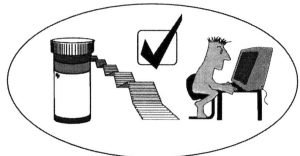

owner's organization, and inspections by regulatory authorities or other external bodies. The *IEEE Standard Glossary of Software Engineering Terminology* gives the following definitions for these three procedures:[1]

- **Audit:** An independent examination of a work product or set of work products to assess compliance with specifications, standards, contractual agreements, or other criteria

- **Inspection:** A static analysis technique that relies on visual examination of development products to detect errors, violations of development standards, and other problems

- **Review:** A process or meeting during which a work product, or set of work products, is

---

1. IEEE Standard Glossary of Software Engineering Terminology—Std. 610.12-1990 (The Institute for Electrical and Electronics Engineers, Inc., Piscataway, NJ, 1986), pp. 11, 40, 64.

presented to project personnel, managers, users, customers, or other interested parties for comment or approval

The objective of an audit is to assess compliance to company policy and relevant regulations. The objective of an inspection is to detect errors, violations, or other problems as measured by external standards. The objective of a system review is to get comment or approval for the system from its internal constituency. The combined experience of all three provides a thorough examination of any system *validation package* and exercises the organization's inspection response model (Figure 9.2).

Whatever model is developed for inspections can also be used for audits and reviews to give participants practice in responding to queries of the *validation package*. An Inspection Response Team (IRT) will be more relaxed and at ease

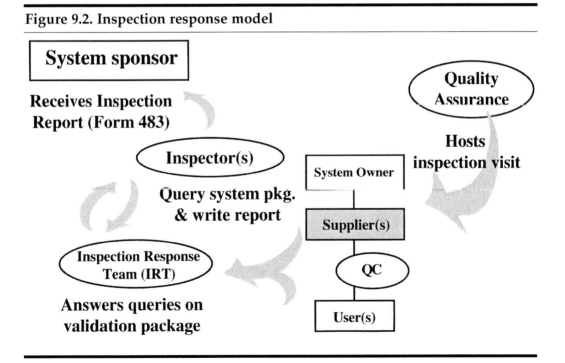

Figure 9.2. Inspection response model

168   The Survive and Thrive Guide to Computer Validation

in dealing with official inspections if its members have already been faced with questions by an audit or review exercise. Practice builds confidence in the team and reinforces confidence in the system.

II. System Owner and System Team Discussion

When a *system owner* and *system team* have worked with a C.V. Policy and Systems QA Plan (SQAP) to develop the appropriate standard system package for their strategic GXP system, they are well placed to welcome a review, audit, or inspection of their system. An independent examination of the system package resulting in a positive report then becomes a reward for their work and a record of achievement to the *system sponsor*. Any comments or suggestions for improvement of the package becomes reinforcement of the good work already performed and establishes a stronger base for system quality and for the next inspection.

While the *system owner* usually initiates a review process and may request a QA audit of the system as part of *validation package* preparation, inspections by external authorities can often come unannounced. With the U.S. FDA, one of the following reasons will initiate an on-site inspection:

- Preapproval inspection of GLP/GCP data handling before granting market authorization for a new product (devices, biologics, drugs).

- Preapproval inspection of a GMP production facility before start of new product manufacture.

- For cause inspection due to problems with data, product safety, or processing quality for a specific product.

- Planned inspection for biennial review (devices, drugs) or for postapproval monitoring of GMP compliance, fraud in the approval process, adverse reaction reporting, or other complaints.

The *system sponsor* and *owner* have a right to know the reason for the inspection visit and can answer queries with

Survive and Thrive with Reviews, Audits, and Inspections   **169**

a better perspective when they understand why the questions are being asked. If the issue is production of a certain product, then the application systems used for that product are fair targets for queries. Other systems are then out of the scope of the inspection and need not be discussed.

Standards for Examination Exercises

There should always be a clear set of standards established as the benchmark for any review, audit, or inspection exercise. General fishing expeditions are not allowed, as they waste time and resources to no specific purpose. The standards can be from regulatory sources, such as those discussed in Chapter 8, or they can be from other industry sources, such as ISO 9000-3, IEEE, or other quality organizations.

For audits and management reviews, the standards used are the organization's own C.V. Policy, SOPs, and any SQAP that may apply. For inspections by a regulatory authority, it is usually the authority's own standards, such as GLP, GCP, or GMP, that provide the benchmark used for the inspection. The inspector will use the GXP regulation as the standard against which to judge the adequacy and completeness of a C.V. Policy, system SOPs, and/or SQAP. System work based on concepts from international standards such as ISO and IEEE are usually recognized by all authorities and can form a common foundation for validation assessment.

If the FDA were to inspect a computerized system used for managing batch records under GMP, laboratory records under GLP, or clinical study records under GCP, the standard it would apply would be 21 CFR 11 Final Rule for Electronic Records and Electronic Signatures.[2] In this regulation example (Figure 9.3), the FDA describes what needs to be done to ensure validation without being precise about how to accomplish the task.

---

2. 21 CFR Part 11—Electronic Records; Electronic Signatures. *Federal Register, Rules and Regulations.* Thursday, March 20, 1997, 62 (54): 13464–13466.

170   The Survive and Thrive Guide to Computer Validation

Figure 9.3. FDA Final Rule—Controls for Electronic Records Systems

. . . systems to create, modify, maintain, or transmit electronic records shall employ procedures and controls designed to ensure the authenticity, integrity, and, when appropriate, the confidentiality of electronic records, and to ensure that the signer cannot readily repudiate the signed record as not genuine. Such procedures and controls shall include the following:

(a)   Validation of systems to ensure accuracy, reliability, consistent intended performance, and the ability to discern invalid or altered records.

(b)   The ability to generate accurate and complete copies of records in both human readable and electronic form suitable for inspection, review, and copying by the agency.

(c)   Protection of records to enable their accurate and ready retrieval throughout the records retention period.

(d)   Limiting system access to authorized individuals.

(e)   Use of secure, computer-generated, time-stamped audit trails to independently record the date and time of operator entries and actions that create, modify, or delete electronic records. Record changes shall not obscure previously recorded information. Such audit trail documentation shall be retained for a period at least as long as that required for the subject electronic records and shall be available for agency review and copying.

(f)   Use of operational system checks to enforce permitted sequencing of steps and events, as appropriate.

(g)   Use of authority checks to ensure that only authorized individuals can use the system, electronically sign a record, access the operation or computer system input or output device, alter a record, or perform the operation at hand.

(h)   Use of device (e.g., terminal) checks to determine, as appropriate, the validity of the source of data input or operational instruction.

(i)   Determination that persons who develop, maintain, or use electronic record/electronic signature systems have the education, raining, and experience to perform their assigned tasks.

(j)   The establishment of, and adherence to, written policies that hold individuals accountable and responsible for actions initiated under their electronic signatures, in order to deter record and signature falsification.

(k)   Use of appropriate controls over system documentation including:

    (1)   Adequate controls over the distribution of, access to, and use of documentation for system operation and maintenance.

    (2)   Revision and change control procedures to maintain an audit trail that documents time-sequenced development and modification of systems documentation.

Survive and Thrive with Reviews, Audits, and Inspections   **171**

Validation of systems, protection of records, and limiting system access are statements that give *system owners* and *system teams* considerable flexibility for how to achieve the desired result. It will be up to the *system owner* and Inspection Response Team to present the *validation package* in a way which shows that inspector how these regulatory requirements have been met.

One way to accomplish this might be to present items from the system package that directly correspond to the list of controls in a regulation. The following list corresponds by letter to the regulation in Figure 9.3.

a. Validation Summary Report

b. Backup and Recovery SOP, example test script and Result Log for checking the retrieval capability of the system

c. Archive management SOP

d. System security SOP, user access and privilege process

e. Description of audit trail function in system manual

f. User SOPs for e-signatures and e-record privileges

g. Test script and Result Log for challenging authority checks of system privileges for different types of users

It is probable that an inspector will be thinking about systems from the perspective of a particular set of GXP regulations. The *system owner* can also consider the same point of view, and, based on the priorities of the relevant regulation(s), can look at the *validation package* and be prepared to select specific evidence to illustrate system quality in terms familiar to the inspector.

Some inspectors do not want a presentation but prefer to dig through documentation on their own. It is still within the *system owner's* and Response Team's control to be sure that relevant items of evidence are provided for inspection review. Since some testing documentation is likely to be examined, the owner can make sure that the scripts initially available include those showing the systems response for priority issues in the regulation. The same priority can be given for providing examples of system and user SOPs.

172 The Survive and Thrive Guide to Computer Validation

Walk-Through Review Process

A walk-through review is an analysis technique in which the *system owner* and IRT lead a review team of interested parties through a description of the system and its operation and the *validation package* of documentation supporting the system. The Walk-Through Team is usually composed of representatives of management, the QA organization, the IT department, and the user community independent of the *system team*. The Walk-Through Team participants ask questions and make comments about possible errors, violation of policy, noncompliance to regulations, and other problems they see based on their view as manager, QA, system user(s), technical support, or other role.

Sometimes the walk-through process is used at the start of a validation activity to develop a baseline assessment of the system prior to working on its *validation package*. In such a case, the Walk-Through Team may include prospective members of a *system team* who use the walk-through process to get to know the system and better understand the gaps to be filled. After the system package is developed, a follow-up walk-through may be conducted with an independent team to review and evaluate the adequacy of the system's package.

In any case, the walk-through process (Figure 9.4) is a formal review of the system's operations, documentation, and intended functions. It often includes a physical tour of the system in its business process and interviews with system users as they work with the system. A designated recorder keeps minutes of Team discussions and drafts a Walk-Through Report with Gap Analysis for Team review and approval.

Walk-Through Preparation and Activity

In preparing for a walk-through review, the *system owner* selects a Walk-Through Team and provides all participants with a premeeting study package. The study package includes a brief description of the system, relevant regulatory

Survive and Thrive with Reviews, Audits, and Inspections   **173**

Figure 9.4. Walk-through review process

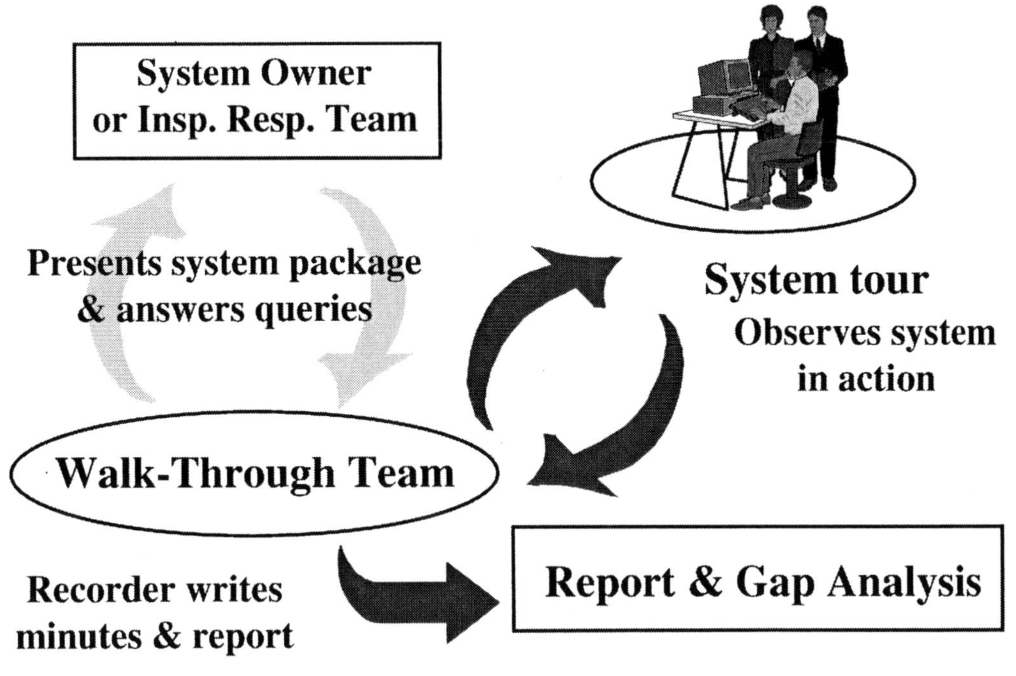

System Owner or Insp. Resp. Team

Presents system package & answers queries

Walk-Through Team

System tour
Observes system in action

Recorder writes minutes & report

Report & Gap Analysis

directives, C.V. Policy, list of relevant SOPs, associated SQAP, and any other standards to be used as benchmarks. The objectives for the walk-through should also be clearly written and provided in the study package. During the walk-through meeting, the following activities take place:

- **System overview:** *System owner* makes an overview presentation of the system under examination and discusses its GXP compliance relevance.

- **Walk-through discussion:** *System owner* leads the team through specific system functions and life cycle documentation so that team members can ask questions and raise issues.

- **Recorded minutes:** A designated recorder minutes all comments and decisions for inclusion in the Walk-Through and Gap Analysis Reports.

174   The Survive and Thrive Guide to Computer Validation

- **Walking tour:** Depending on the size and complexity of the system(s) being examined, the Walk-Through Team may decide to conduct a physical walking tour that traces the whole process using the computerized system(s) and includes observing the system(s) in operation.

During a physical walking tour of the system in operation, the Walk-Through Team performs the following activities:

- Records all points of electronic data capture, process control, automated calculations, interactions with other systems, data transfer, or other GXP related activity performed by the system

- Evaluates each electronic point for its Safety, Efficacy, and Quality (SEQ) impact on GXP data and regulated product

- Identifies any human checkpoints for controlling system performance

- Notes environmental conditions and hazards

- Checks user materials available in the operating environment for accuracy, completeness, and up-to-date content with approval signatures and dates

- Asks users to explain how they operate the system, report problems, seek help, and fix the system to see if they understand and adhere to SOPs

- Observes backup and archival tapes for system and data and checks for conformance to system SOP procedures

- Examines the interaction between the system and the GXP process it supports for unintended use of the system by operator workarounds to solve problems in performance or new requirements in the process not incorporated in the original system design

Walk-Through Report and Gap Analysis

Upon completion of the walk-through meeting and physical walking tour, the team may recommend a follow-up meeting to set priorities and build a consensus for how to

Survive and Thrive with Reviews, Audits, and Inspections 175

proceed to bring the system(s) into better compliance with GXP regulations. All "gaps" or missing elements in compliance readiness of the system are assessed for their SEQ impact and assigned a priority based upon SEQ and other risk, hazard or criticality measurements established by local SOPs or the team as a group.

Within a reasonable time after the walk-through, the recorder issues a Walk-Through Report detailing the findings for the *system owner.* This report contains the following items:

- Identification of the walk-through team members
- Identification of the system(s) being examined
- Statement of the objectives to be handled during the walk-through including the regulations and other standards used as benchmarks for the system review
- A prioritized list of noted deficiencies, omissions, issues, and suggestions for improvement
- Any recommendations made by the walk-through team to close the "gaps," fix deficiencies, and resolve issues
- If follow-up walk-through reviews are suggested, then this is also in the report.

The Walk-Through Report, meeting minutes, and any other materials used as a basis for conclusions should be included in system documentation files and stored as per local QA SOP. The details of the report usually remain company confidential, but a record is made in the system's Configuration Management Logbook that a walk-through was conducted on a specific date and a report was issued on a specific date. When the recommendations are acted on by the *system owner,* an appropriate log entry is made for actions taken.

Benefits of a Walk-Through and Gap Analysis

System owners receive many benefits form experiencing a walk-through exercise. It forces them to organize their *validation package* materials in a coherent way and to develop a logical presentation of what the system is, how it operates, and how it fits into the GXP process it supports. Having the views of other people with an independent perspective on the system can bring out weaknesses that the *owner* would not have considered because he or she always thinks of the system in a single, familiar way.

Discussing and defending the system and its documentation against the standards being applied by the Walk-Through Team members stretches the awareness of the *system owner* for other interpretations of the benchmarks. The walk-through meetings and physical tour can also be used to prepare and train for a logical approach to future audits and inspections.

SOP for Systems Audit or Inspection

Every organizational site subject to a systems audit or inspection should have an SOP to follow for how such an experience is to be handled. Every strategic system subject to audit or inspection should have at least one query response person plus a backup response person assigned and trained in presenting the contents of the system's *validation package.* In addition, on a per site basis, a quality professional should be assigned to greet an external auditor or inspector and serve as host in support of the official review visit.

The role of host should have its duties specified. Such duties should include at least the following:

- Greet the auditor or inspector and escort him or her to an appropriate conference room for use as an office and base of operation during their stay.

- Identify the purpose and scope of the audit or inspection and the specific objectives for this visit. A general faultfinding expedition is not allowed. The exercise should be product or problem-specific or part of contract negotiations to assess capabilities for performing certain services.

Survive and Thrive with Reviews, Audits, and Inspections   177

- Notify appropriate management, quality, and systems people of the arrival of the auditor or inspector and the purpose of their visit.

- Hold an opening session to plan for *system owner* meetings and documentation review for target systems.

- If a tour of the facility is requested, arrange one, and accompany the auditor or inspector on the tour.

- Attend all meetings and record all discussion points brought up by the auditor or inspector.

- Retain a duplicate copy of any document copied for the auditor or inspector. When in doubt about site confidentiality issues, check with QA director before showing or releasing a document to the auditor or inspector. Only documents that are related to the purpose and objective of the inspection are subject to review.

- Ensure that the auditor or inspector is escorted at all times while on the premises. Casual conversations overheard in the cafeteria or rest room can introduce unintended topics into the inspection focus.

- Be truthful when responding to queries on *validation packages*, and be comfortable with saying, "I don't know" when that is the case.

- Organize a final wrap-up meeting to hear the auditor or inspector's preliminary findings.

- Hold a debriefing session after the audit or inspection is concluded to assess comments, concerns, and knowledge gained by all participants in the experience.

- Write up a hosting report for management review to include all activities observed, people interviewed, documents copied, systems examined, and concerns or suggestions expressed by the auditor or inspector.

System owners participating in an audit/inspection interview should be prepared to give a brief description of their system and be able to present the contents of the system's *validation package* in a logical way. They should be familiar with the organization's C.V. Policy and any general SOP (GOP), local SOP, or SQAP relevant to the system so that the auditor or inspector understands the context in which the package has been developed (Figure 9.5).

A *system owner* should be able to discuss and defend the contents of a system's standard package and the strategy behind the development of the package, whether it is prospective, retrospective or verification of a newly developed system. Nothing impresses an auditor more than to interview a *system owner* who has all his or her *validation package* documentation out on the table ready for review and who is ready to map a logical path through the material at hand.

It is especially important to understand and be able to discuss the testing strategy and Test Summary Report for a system. Configuration management and the logbooks that record system management activities are also very important components of the package. Training records are usually the stepchild of any *validation package,* and some thought should be given to having examples of such training documentation available for review.

Figure 9.5. System package in context

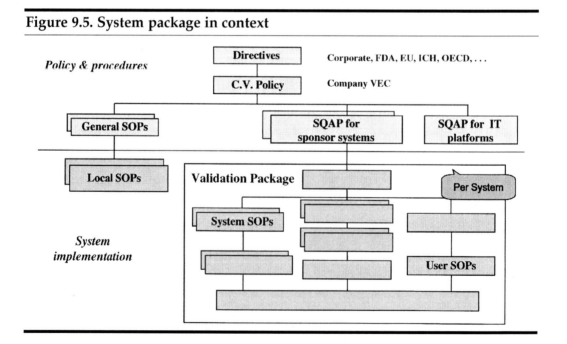

Survive and Thrive with Reviews, Audits, and Inspections

Internal and external suppliers of GXP software and systems should also be ready to discuss and defend their *verification package* for the SDLC. Vendor audits by prospective customers as well as inspections by authorities are a business requirement for GXP systems and should be negotiated and planned for in a formal way by *system owners* at the time of acquisition.

Follow-up Actions to Audits and Inspections

In addition to the Hosting Report, the *system owner* should receive an Audit or Inspection Report. The U.S. FDA inspectors write their observations on an FDA 483 form. Auditors will have other formats. While inspections often focus on errors and omissions, an Audit Report should include both site strengths and site weaknesses. The benchmark used to determine strength or weakness should be specified at the beginning of the report.

All audits and inspections should use an external standard for measurement, and while there is always an element of experience-based interpretation of a standard, the Audit/ Inspection Report should not be founded on personal opinion. *System owners* and IRTs should not, however, get into an emotional discussion with any auditor or inspector about technical issues. Be prepared to base your *validation package* approach on points that can be traced to or adapted from international standards and regulatory documents.

The *system owner* is expected to review the audit or inspection findings with management and QA and to implement a Way Forward Plan to address issues and concerns raised about the system. The final report from an auditor or inspector should include items as discussed during interviews or at the wrap-up session. There should be no major surprises coming after the visit wrap-up discussion.

When follow-up action is taken to an Audit or Inspection Report, it should be recorded in appropriate System Logs. Within four to six months of receiving an Audit/Inspection Report, a *system owner* should be able to write a report to management, citing the log entries or other documents that record the actions taken to address specific items cited in the Audit/Inspection Report. Such a follow-up report should also discuss the rationale for items not addressed and give a Way Forward Plan as necessary for more extensive follow-up work. As with all reports, plans, and validation documents, *brevity is beautiful,* and a minimum number of pages is the goal for direct communication of specific information.

Regulatory Consequences for Inspection Issues

The business consequences of regulatory concerns from inspections vary from country to country, depending on local laws. In the United States, the FDA has three levels of action open to it. The first action is always a written Form 483 made by the inspectors to record observations made during their visit. If serious concerns are observed, a warning letter may be sent to the company to cite the concerns and give a specific time limit for addressing the concerns and for a return of the inspectors to see how the concerns have been fixed.

If warning letters do not produce the needed corrective actions, then a court ruling or injunction can follow. For GMP violations, the court could authorize seizure of a product or injunction against further production that prevents the company from shipping product. For GLP or GCP violations, action can be taken to deny submission of study data for pivotal trials or toxicology studies where system integrity is in question. This would require redoing clinical trials or animal studies and result in a greatly increased cost and time for bringing a new drug to market. Such cost would be considerably higher than the effort required to have a solid *validation package* in place to begin with. In cases of fraudulent data and practices, convictions have resulted in senior managers serving jail sentences and physicians being disbarred from conducting clinical trials.

Survive and Thrive with Reviews, Audits, and Inspections   **181**

III. Conclusion

Pride in System Performance

Objective grounds for an *owner's* pride in system performance is illustrated in the standard *validation packages* shown in Chapters 3–5. These packages provide a clear view of the quality of a computerized system. *System teams* can take pride in developing them and keeping them up-to-date, for they are the health record of the system and the windows through which auditors and inspectors review the system. This chapter discusses a walk-through review process to help owners prepare for audits and inspections of strategic systems, so that they can use the *validation packages* to answer the general checklist of questions shown in Figure 9.6.[3]

Companies and sites that invest in computerized systems want them to work right and expect their data handling activities to give reliable information that is protected from loss or harm. Auditors and inspectors have the same goals —reliable systems and protected data integrity. Chapters 2–8 present a standards-based approach to ensuring management control, data integrity, and system reliability with documented evidence to make the quality auditable.

---

3. T. Stokes, Computer Systems Validation, Part 6: A Survive and Thrive Approach to Audits and Inspections. *Applied Clinical Trials* (August 1997): 40–44.

182   The Survive and Thrive Guide to Computer Validation

Figure 9.6. General checklist for audits and inspections

In general, for a GXP system, the system owner should have documented evidence in response to the following dozen questions:

1. What does this system do and how was it developed?

2. How was the system tested and accepted for operational use? When was it last tested?

3. How are people trained on the system? How is training recorded?

4. Does the system environment meet supplier's specifications?

5. Is the system serviced and maintained at regular intervals? Are there records?

6. What are the backup and recovery procedures for hardware, software, data, and communications?

7. Are there alternative arrangements for disaster recovery in case of flood, fire, or theft? Have they been exercised?

8. How is physical and logical security provided for the system? Who is authorized to enter and/or edit data? Are electronic signatures used?

9. How are problems reported and handled for user and technical support issues?

10. How are changes managed for the system and its components? Who authorizes changes? What records are kept?

11. With what other systems does this system communicate or transfer data? How is this controlled and monitored for quality of interaction?

12. Has this system been audited before? Were follow-up actions taken? When was the last audit or inspection?

10. Laboratory Systems

I. System Sponsor's Summary

There are countless configurations of computerized instruments and data handling units used in the modern laboratory today (Figure 10.1). The simplest of these is the automated instrument with a digital readout. The next level is the multichannel instrument with a dedicated personal computer to control it. Then there is the data system

Figure 10.1. Laboratory view—computer system

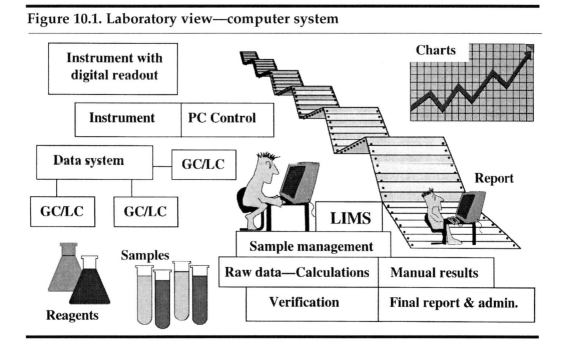

184   The Survive and Thrive Guide to Computer Validation

that collects and processes output from more than one instrument, such as a chromatography data system collecting data from multiple gas or liquid chromatographic (GC/LC) instruments. The final step is the laboratory-wide information management system (LIMS) that manages samples; schedules testing; assigns personnel and instruments; receives data from both manual and automated sources; calculates and reports final results; provides audit trails of data changes; and archives lab data, final reports, and administrative information.

Automation and LIMS—Good Automated Laboratory Practice (GALP)

Organizations that rely on laboratory results to accomplish their mission have come to recognize the importance of computers as an equal partner in the analysis process and look to validation of the computerized elements as an important component of the overall suitability testing of automated instrumentation. The U.S. Environmental Protection Agency (EPA) relies on laboratory data from its own and independent analytical laboratories in order to administer its various regulatory responsibilities. In 1995, it published an update to its guideline for Good Automated Laboratory Practices, known as the GALPs. This document recognizes the complexity of computerized laboratory operations and finds it helpful to think of all laboratory computer configurations as one of two categories—LIMS and non-LIMS.[1]

GALP Definitions:

- **LIMS:** automated laboratory systems that collect and manage data. This includes most configurations that are involved with entering, recording, manipulating, modifying, and retrieving data.

- **Non-LIMS:** automated laboratory systems that record data, but do not allow changes to the data are not LIMS.

---

1. *Good Automated Laboratory Practices: Principles and Guidance to Regulations for Ensuring Data Integrity in Automated Laboratory Operations with Implementation Guidance* (U.S. Environmental Protection Agency. Research Triangle Park, NC. 1995), pp. 1-2, 1-3.

An instrument that measures weights and produces or maintains a readout of the weight is not a LIMS if the true reading cannot be altered by a person prior to recording.

The ability to effect changes to original observations is the factor that determines whether an automated laboratory system is a LIMS. If data entering automated laboratory systems can be manipulated or changed in any way by the action of a person prior to being recorded, then that automated system is a LIMS.

The principles of the GALP regulation and guidance are shown on the matrix in Figure 10.2. *System sponsors* will recognize familiar concepts from OECD GLP and EU Annex 11.

With the GALP, as with all the other regulatory directives, management continues to carry final responsibility for the integrity of data submitted to regulatory authorities. The fact that data have become electronic does not remove

Figure 10.2. Principles of EPA GALP for LIMS

Management control	**System reliability**
a. Management method(s) to ensure integrity of all LIMS data e. User SOPs, training, and support documentation	d. Change controls for LIMS operations and software f. Backup, recovery, and disaster recovery SOPs
Data integrity	**Auditable quality**
c. Audit trail for LIMS raw data entry, change, and recording	b. LIMS formulas and decision algorithms must be inspected and verified

186   The Survive and Thrive Guide to Computer Validation

management's role and give it to the IT Department. Electronic data just add an electronic dimension to management's domain and require policy and procedures to ensure data integrity and system reliability with training and follow-up audits to monitor compliance.

II. System Owner and System Team Discussion

The EU GMP Guide Annex 11 gives the laboratory analyst a quick, concise, four-page overview of system concepts for good practice, and the OECD GLP Consensus Document adds 14 more pages of details that are relevant to laboratory studies. The EPA GALP document, however, goes a large step further by providing an implementation chapter with 130 pages of guidance to help *system owners* and *system teams* understand just how to go about installing Good Automated Laboratory Practices in any laboratory situation.

Step 1: Walk-Through Review, Systems Inventory, and Gap Analysis

Use the GALP's broad-based definition of LIMS to identify all computerized systems in the laboratory that are candidates for validation. This can be done by conducting a walk-through of the laboratory by a team consisting of the laboratory supervisor, the QA auditor for the lab, and an IT professional. Analysts responsible for the automation systems in the lab would then be interviewed in situ about their systems. The availability of SOPs and logbooks and documentation at the lab bench can then be observed and their condition assessed.

This initial review walk-through is expected to develop an annotated inventory of LIMS systems with a preliminary analysis of any obvious gaps between their current status and the requirements of good practice stated in OECD GLP and EPA GALP. The walk-through discussions introduce the validation concepts to all the analysts interviewed and the walk-through report provides a baseline picture of lab systems to keep reality in focus during the development of a Systems QA Plan (SQAP) for the laboratory.

Step 2: SQAP Development and Policy Statement

The first agenda for the SQAP Team is to examine the organization's C.V. Policy in light of the baseline walk-through experience. Any adaptations or modifications required for the laboratory situation can the be included in a policy statement that lab management can review and approve. Items such as the definition and use of Safety, Efficacy, and Quality (SEQ) analysis may be one area for adaptation.

As discussed in Chapter 6, an SQAP can be developed to give guidance to all personnel involved in systems validation activities. The size and scope of effort for different types of automation in the lab can be described and templates provided to make the work easier and more consistent across different systems. The rationale behind both the Policy and SQAP is stated very well by the six principles of the GALP (Figure 10.3).[2]

The SQAP should provide guidance and support for *System teams* working to apply each of the six principles to their laboratory systems.

Step 3: Standard Operating Procedures

Laboratory management is expected to ensure that SOPs are reviewed periodically to check that they accurately describe the current system procedures. Management authorizes each SOP and any subsequent changes to the SOP. Previous versions of LIMS SOPs are retained in an historical file.

Both the EPA GALP and the OECD GLP provide listings of a basic set of SOPs for good practice with laboratory

---

2. GALP, pp. 2-1, 2-2.

188 The Survive and Thrive Guide to Computer Validation

Figure 10.3. Six principles for LIMS quality—EPA GALP 1995

a. **Laboratory management must provide a method of assuring the integrity of all LIMS data.**

Communication, transfer, manipulation, and the storage/recall process all offer potential for data corruption. The demonstration of control necessitates the collection of evidence to prove that the system provides reasonable protection against data corruption.

b. **The formulas and decision algorithms employed by the LIMS must be accurate and appropriate.**

Users cannot assume that the test or decision criteria are correct; those formulas must be inspected and verified.

c. **A critical control element is the capability to track LIMS Raw Data entry, modification, and recording to the responsible person.**

This capability utilizes a password system or equivalent to identify the time, date, and person or persons entering, modifying, or recording data.

d. **Consistent and appropriate change controls, capable of tracking the LIMS operations and software, are a vital element in the control process.**

All changes must follow carefully planned procedures, be properly documented, and, when appropriate, include acceptance testing.

e. **Procedures must be established and documented for all users to follow. Control of even the most carefully designed and implemented LIMS will be thwarted if the user does not follow these procedures.**

This principle implies the development of clear directions and SOP; the training of all users, and the availability of appropriate user support documentation.

f. **The risk of LIMS failure requires that procedures be established and documented to minimize and manage their occurrences.**

Where appropriate, redundant systems must be installed and periodic system backups must be performed at a frequency consistent with the consequences of the loss of information resulting from failure. The principle of control must extend to planning for reasonable unusual events and system stresses.

---

systems. The GALP list of basic SOPs (Figure 10.4) is a useful guide for establishing general operating procedures to be applied across the laboratory, and the OECD GLP list (Figure 4.11) can be applied to specific systems and their *validation packages*.[3]

Laboratory Systems **189**

Figure 10.4. Basic set of SOPs—EPA GALP 1995

1.	Identification and documentation of LIMS raw rata and LIMS raw data storage
2.	Verification of LIMS raw data
3.	Changes to LIMS raw data
4.	Software development methodologies
5.	Software testing and quality assurance
6.	Software change control
7.	Software version control
8.	Software historical file
9.	Hardware changes
10.	Hardware testing, inspection, and maintenance
11.	Records retention

Step 4: Assign Teams and Develop System Packages

When the baseline inventory of systems has been prioritized according to the SQAP guidelines, *system owners* are assigned and validation system work begins. The EPA GALP recommends essentially the same life cycle approach as the one described in Chapter 2. It describes the complete software life cycle to include the phases of initiation, requirements analysis, design, programming, testing and quality assurance, installation and operation, maintenance and enhancement, and retirement. All phases of the life cycle are to be documented in a way that is consistent with the size and scope of the system, the sensitivity of the data it handles, and the diversity of organizations using the system.

The appropriate standard system *validation packages* as described in Chapters 3–5 are then developed under the direction of the *system owners*. Most professionally run

---

3. GALP, p. 2-122.

laboratories have a very tight system of quality control for the analytical procedure that uses automated instrumentation. This analytical QC can often be used as one form of "black box" testing of the computerized component. Standard reagent samples with known values that are run through the analytical process and yield their expected standard values in the computerized component provide ongoing testing support for data integrity and system reliability. They cannot, however, do the whole job of exercising and stressing all the key functions of the computerized system.

Step 5: Use a Standard Laboratory Data Handling Model

Although instrumentation and methods may vary, there is a basic view of electronic data handling as shown in Figure 10.5 that is much the same regardless of the specialty or location of the laboratory. A QC laboratory analyzing raw

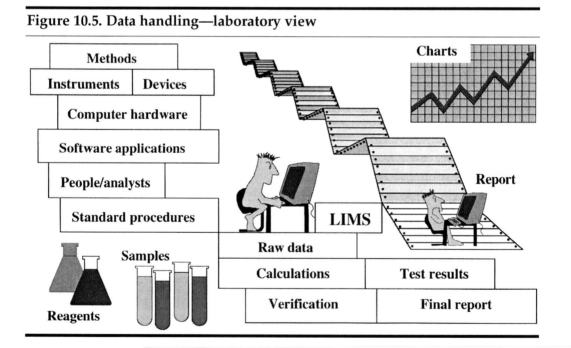

Figure 10.5. Data handling—laboratory view

Laboratory Systems   191

materials or finished product at a manufacturing site, a clinical laboratory processing patient samples in a hospital, or a toxicology lab studying animal specimens all use the same model.

All laboratory analyses operate with specific methods that analysts perform using written standard procedures. The analyses employ various instruments and devices that are automated with computer hardware and software applications to produce raw data. In an instrument-based LIMS or a data station LIMS or in a laboratory-wide LIMS, the raw data undergoes specific calculations, modifications, or transformations to give test results. The test results are checked and verified, and then a final analytical report is released.

For the final report to be acceptable, the analytical process must be performed correctly and the computerized data handling in the LIMS must be accurate. Identification of the analyst and the time and date of the testing are also recorded with the raw data and final result to provide an "audit trail" for future reference. Any change made to raw data or the final result must be included as an "add-on" to the audit trail with a reason for the change included and the original result retained for historical review during audit and inspection.

It is logical to assume that the size and scope of the validation effort in support of the six GALP principles will depend on the complexity of the various LIMS systems to be found in a particular laboratory. When management develops a C.V. Policy or SQAP for the laboratory, it can define categories of automation and the level of attention to be given per level.

Whenever possible, the ongoing quality control efforts of the laboratory for its analytical methods should be partnered with the validation efforts for its computer automation. If known standards are used to calibrate the analytical procedure every time a particular test is performed, then the calibration of the automation used in the analysis may be a byproduct of the same effort. The Test Plan for such an automated instrument could then cite the standards testing

The Survive and Thrive Guide to Computer Validation

as part of its ongoing validation testing and an element in its *validation package*.

Step 6: Establish Instrument Automation Logbooks

Every automated instrument should have a bound logbook associated with it. Usually this logbook records all calibration, maintenance, and QC activities performed on the instrument as well as the daily operational notes of the analyst. Such a logbook also needs to include a validation section for the computerized components associated with the instrument.

The Automation Logbook would include sections for recording the following issues:

- **Shift Report**—an analyst's Shift Report for any unexpected events occurring

- **Problem Report**—problem tracking and resolution log

- **HW Changes**—change control log for hardware components

- **SW Changes**—change control for system and application software

- **Testing**—Testing Log for checking the automation control and data handling capabilities

- **Maintenance**—log for calibration and maintenance of hardware and software

- **Audits**—log of the dates of QC reviews, QA audits, and inspections of the system

- **Documentation**—reference section to identify relevant SOPs, manuals, and other laboratory documents or *validation package* items associated with the instrument

The Automation Logbook is not a replacement for a standard *validation package*. It is an ongoing support mechanism for the *validation package* and should be prescribed in the Validation Plan. The process for developing standard system *validation packages* in the laboratory is the same as

Laboratory Systems   **193**

for any other area of the organization and has been described in Chapters 3–5.

Step 7: Document Legacy Automation Systems

It is not unusual for a laboratory to have computerized instrumentation on-line over time (legacy system) that has never had its automation fully described and validated. In other cases, several instruments may have been connected together with computerized elements to accomplish specific analytical purposes and never documented. If management designates such a system as a validation priority, it must have a system description as a starter to any *validation package*. Experience has shown that in such cases the procedure described in Figure 10.6 can be a practical approach.

This process maps three paths through the procedure. The first path is the familiar one of analyst and instrument activities required by the analytical process. The second path identifies every point of electronic interaction with the automation system such as data entry, change, or retrieval by keyboard, wand, stylus, or other automated device. The third path describes the LIMS data handling response to each electronic point of interaction as in Figure 10.6 and adds in any calculations or transformations of data occurring between or during analytical steps.

SOPs and System User Manuals should be used to support the walk-through. Check to see if they are up-to-date with how the analysts currently perform the procedure. It is important to have the analyst demonstrate with an actual run of samples and not just talk about how a lab test is performed. Often with legacy systems, there are adjustments made and workarounds employed that become so automatic that analysts don't think to mention them, they are not written down anywhere, and they could involve electronic points and LIMS operations.

Once the three paths have been completed, a description of the key functions of the legacy automation system has been

194   The Survive and Thrive Guide to Computer Validation

Figure 10.6. Describing a Legacy Automation System

Perform a walk-through of the analytical procedure using the system and note the following:

1—Analytical Steps	2—Electronic Points	3—LIMS Data Operations
1. Wand sample and fill instrument cup	1. Bar code reading	1. Link bar code ID with cup ID to identify sample

---

developed. This description then becomes a part of the standard system *validation package* and can form a realistic basis for Validation Plan strategies and Test Plan approaches to the system. From the OECD perspective, any GLP application description should have documentation with the following information:[4]

- The name of the application software or identification code and a detailed and clear description of the purpose of the application

- The hardware (with model numbers) on which the application software operates

- The operating system and other system software (e.g., tools) used in conjunction with the application

- The application programming language(s) and/or data base tools used

- The major functions performed by the application

- An overview of the type and flow of data/data base design associated with the application

---

4. *GLP Consensus Document: The Application of the Principles of GLP to Computerized Systems*, Environment Monograph No. 116 (Environment Directorate, OECD, Paris, 1995), Section 8b.

- File structures, error and alarm message, and algorithms associated with the application

- The application software components with version numbers

- Configuration and communication links among application modules and to equipment and other systems

Step 8: Plan for Electronic Records Retention and System Retirement

Both the OECD GLP and EPA GALP documents require that SOPs be established in the laboratory for change control of raw data and for managing the retention of electronic raw data on media that keep it accessible for the regulated storage time. Both documents also require that sufficient physical, logical, and backup security measures be taken to ensure the integrity of electronic data over time.

In Section 9, the OECD GLP Consensus Document gives more detailed directives about managing records in archives, and it stresses that electronic data be stored with the same levels of access control, indexing, and expedient retrieval as other types of data. Where electronic data from more than one study is stored on a single medium, such as a disk or tape, a detailed index is required. The OECD acknowledges that special facilities with specific environmental controls may be required for archiving electronic data and recommends that personnel be assigned for managing such facilities and that access to such facilities be limited to authorized personnel only.

When computerized systems are to be retired, the OECD requires that procedures be exercised to provide continued readability of the data. This could be accomplished by transferring the data to another system or by making hard copy printouts. No electronically stored data are to be destroyed without management approval and relevant documentation. Other data about the computerized systems such as source code and records for development,

196   The Survive and Thrive Guide to Computer Validation

validation, operation, maintenance, and monitoring are to be held for at least as long as the study records associated with the systems.

The basic message from both GLP and GALP is that it is very important to plan carefully for the managed care of archived data and the continued accessibility of data from retiring systems. Phase 9 of the systems life cycle, "Retirement and Replacement," is just as important as Phase 1. Most regulated laboratories have a system in place for the archival of paper records, but some need to be reminded that equal focus must now be given to archiving electronic records and the documentation associated with electronic systems.

The electronic records of particular concern are electronic forms of *raw data*. The OECD defines raw data as being

all original laboratory records and documentation, including data directly entered into a computer through an instrument interface, which are the results of original observations and activities in a study and which are necessary for the reconstruction and evaluation of the report of that study.[5]

The EPA GALP defines LIMS raw data as

original observations recorded by the LIMS that are needed to verify, calculate, or derive data that are or may be reported.[6]

The protection of such material can be planned by developing an SOP for managing the electronic records archive (Figure 10.7).

Step 9: Practice for Audits and Inspections

As discussed in Chapter 9, it is a good idea to develop an inspection response model for the laboratory so that people

---

5. GLP, Section 5.

6. GALP, pp. 1–16.

Laboratory Systems   197

Figure 10.7. Electronic records archive management SOP

This SOP provides written procedures to cover the following topics:

- how to label different types of media-diskettes, tapes, CDs, paper, etc.
- how to index and retrieve different types of media
- how to monitor and verify the integrity of stored records
- laboratory retention times for different types of records
- environmental controls for media archives
- security and disaster recovery procedures for media archives
- change control practices for technology and data during:
  - entry and exit of records from the archive
  - entry and exit of media types from the archive
  - entry and exit of systems from the archive
- authorization process for personnel who:
  - manage electronic archives
  - have access to archived records
  - delete archived material after retention period has ended

understand their role and responsibility during audits and inspections. Every system subject to inspection should have a primary response person and a backup response person who know the *validation package* for the system and can answer queries on the package. Users of those systems should also be taught how to conduct themselves when operating the system during an inspection. They should answer questions directly and concisely, and not go into long war stories about how awful things were in the past and how they came along to clean up the mess.

Walk-through reviews of specific systems by laboratory supervisors can provide *system owners* and response teams with an audit-like experience that also gives management a view of the preparedness of the laboratory for GLP inspection. Informal audits by the Quality Assurance Unit (QAU) associated with the laboratory can also provide

198   The Survive and Thrive Guide to Computer Validation

good experience. Any such activities should be noted in the Automation Logbooks by date and name of reviewer, and a confidential written report stating strengths and weaknesses should be prepared and shared with *system owners* for feedback and follow-up action.

III.   Conclusion

Simple Definition and Defined Approach

Given the limitless variety of configurations of computerized systems in today's laboratories, it is important to define validation candidates in the laboratory in a simple way. The EPA GALP does this by applying its directives to all LIMS systems and then defining a LIMS system as one where the ability to effect changes to original observations is the determining factor. If data entering automated laboratory systems can be manipulated or changed in any way by the action of a person prior to being recorded, then that automated system is a LIMS and becomes a candidate for validation.

Various regulatory directives such as the OECD GLP Consensus and EPA GALP have common themes for protecting the integrity of electronic raw data and derived data in the laboratory. Validation of computerized systems is recognized as a necessary activity to ensure the integrity of laboratory data. The system validation practices of Chapters 1–9 can be applied in a straightforward fashion to laboratory situations in order to meet such directives.

11. Clinical Research Systems

I. System Sponsor's Summary

Traditionally, clinical research systems have been considered the computer systems used within a sponsoring company for data management of case report form (CRF) information, for statistical analysis, for tracking serious adverse events (SAEs), and for publishing final reports and new drug applications. As shown in Figure 11.1, these

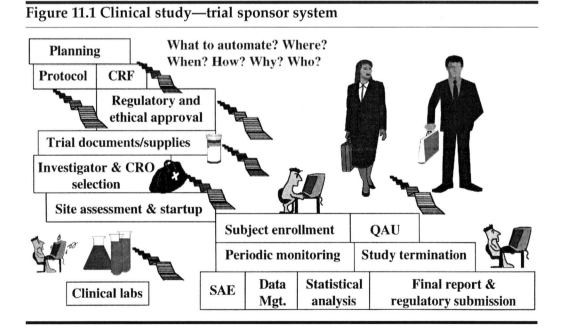

Figure 11.1 Clinical study—trial sponsor system

traditional systems continue to be used as general clinical computing resources across all protocols and studies. They are the first targets for computer *validation package* development.

Today, many other systems are coming into use for GCP activities in the *sponsor's* clinical trial process. Such new systems may include document management systems for SOP distribution and workflow approval of clinical study documents, electronic CRFs (e-CRFs), supply ordering and tracking systems, databases at clinical research organizations (CROs), central laboratories, investigator sites, and laptop systems for trial administration and tracking by clinical research associates (CRAs). *System sponsors* in clinical research need to develop policy and procedures for deciding which systems require standard *validation packages* and which follow other company procedures for systems quality assurance.

Starting with the European GCP in 1992, regulatory authorities have increasingly focused on the integrity of electronic records and the validation of computerized systems used in clinical studies. As discussed in Chapter 8 (Figure 8.13), the ICH GCP has a strong section on the validation of electronic trial data handling systems.

With the practice of modern medicine becoming more and more automated, new categories of computerized systems outside of the trial sponsor's organization can become of GCP concern depending on the requirements of a specific protocol. Sometimes these systems are worn by the subject as monitoring instruments; sometimes they are even inside the patient in the form of medical devices, they are used by subjects as electronic diaries, or they calculate and control delivery of therapy dosages as in various radiation treatments. The ability of such systems to perform as intended can no longer be assumed.

As more and more companies outsource the conduct of their trials to clinical research organizations (CROs) and use central laboratories for analyses, the validation status of systems used in these suppliers becomes a GCP concern. Since the trial sponsor always keeps responsibility for the integrity of GCP data and for the GCP compliance of all studies no matter who conducts them, it is important that trial sponsors can trust the electronic data handling of all contractors supporting clinical research activities, whether they be CROs, laboratories, or investigator sites. The trial sponsor's SOP for supplier management and contract practices needs to include elements for qualifying and auditing computer validation practices and the GCP integrity of electronic data handling performed under contract by external parties.

System Categories—Trial Sponsor and Nonsponsor, GCP and Non-GCP

It is important to sort out validation responsibilities for GCP systems and electronic data (e-data). The developers of the Medical Monitoring Plan and the Data Management Plan need to examine the protocol and identify the types of e-data to be collected, likely sources of electronic raw data, and the kinds of e-data handling systems likely to be used during studies.

The qualifier for GCP focus is data that are used to prove to authorities the safety, efficacy, or quality (SEQ) of regulated product or systems used to control the process of delivering the study therapy. Figure 11.2 shows a matrix for reviewing study protocols and classifying systems used according to their ownership by either the trial sponsor's organization or any of the nonsponsor groups involved in conducting a specific trial and by their GCP or non-GCP status.

A clinical Computer Validation (C.V.) Policy can state that for trial sponsor systems, validation is performed directly by the trial sponsor's organization according to the system's GCP and SEQ priority. For nonsponsor GCP systems, SOP direction is given for the qualification, monitoring and auditing of systems on a per protocol basis as part of the supplier management process for third parties conducting clinical trial activities.

Requiring protocols to develop a matrix map of the types of GCP data systems used for their studies gives early

202   The Survive and Thrive Guide to Computer Validation

Figure 11.2. Protocol matrix of trial data systems

	Trial sponsor systems	Nonsponsor systems
GCP systems	General systems Protocol-specific systems <small>Used in-house</small> <small>Provided to sites</small>	CRO Investigator Lab/hospital Subject
Non-GCP systems	General systems Protocol-specific systems <small>Used in-house</small> <small>Provided to sites</small>	CRO Investigator Lab/hospital Subject

visibility to the issues relevant to e-data integrity and system reliability. These issues can then be addressed as part of the medical monitoring and data management plans and third party contracts for study support. Planning up-front for site qualification, audit, and monitoring activities to support the QA of e-data and GCP systems inspires confidence in the decision-making data and enables trouble-free inspection of pivotal studies.

The matrix analysis approach to GCP systems documents a rationale for action in support of e-data compliance issues. The matrix provides a systems map for addressing the concerns of Section 5.8 of the ICH Draft Guideline on Statistical Principles for Clinical Trials, which states the following:[1]

5.8 Integrity of Data and Computer Software
The credibility of the numerical results of the analysis depends on the quality and validity of the

---

1. International Conference on Harmonization: Draft Guideline on Statistical Principles for Clinical Trials; Notice of Availability. *Federal Register* May 9, 1997 (Volume 62, No. 90), Section 5.8, p. 25723.

methods and software used both for data management (data entry, storage, verification, correction, and retrieval) and for processing the data statistically. Data management activities should therefore be based on thorough and effective SOPs. The computer software used for data management and statistical analysis should be reliable, and documentation of appropriate software testing procedures should be available.

II. System Owner and System Team Discussion

When considering the classification of systems in Figure 11.2, there are two concepts to be discussed by *system owners*. The first is the standard situation that applies to trial sponsor systems classified as GCP relevant, and in this case all the usual practices apply for *system owners* and *system teams* as described in Chapters 1–9. The second concept is the situation of nonsponsor Systems classified as GCP relevant and that reside under the management of third parties.

In the second instance, the trial sponsor company is the *"system sponsor"* responsible for the GCP status of data from contracted third party systems. The CRAs or monitors who qualify and/or contract with the third parties are the *"system owners"* for sites under their supervision. In this case, the *"system team"* is the third party site itself. The CRA/medical monitor has only two ways to ensure e-data and system compliance-by including terms for validation of e-data and GCP systems in the third party contract and by site monitoring and auditing practices.

A Way Forward Plan for GCP computers would start with provisions for validating the traditional general systems in the clinical research organization of the trial sponsor. It would then consider GCP compliance for third-party systems used in a trial and systems deployed by the trial sponsor to third-party sites for study-specific data collection. The general strategy for these three types of systems could be defined in a C.V. Policy for clinical systems and the practical approach discussed in an SQAP for clinical systems.

The six-step discussion that follows is intended to provide guidance for developing a Way Forward Plan.

Step 1: Identify and Validate General Systems at Trial Sponsor Location(s)

As a first priority, the general systems that trial sponsor companies normally target for GCP validation efforts include the CRF data management system, the SAE data management and reporting system, the statistical analysis system, and the tracking system for supplies of study drug or other investigative product. Developing a standard *validation package* for any one of these general systems will suffice to establish that system's use as compliant for all studies.

The development, validation, and use of standard modules for formatting database elements and other configurable items in general systems will reduce the custom work required for specific protocols. This, in turn, will speed the preparation of data handling for a protocol and reduce the need for extra testing and validation work on a per protocol basis. Validation of the GCP general systems used across all trials is the first step for a trial sponsor or CRO in working toward compliance.

Step 2: Identify and Validate Custom-Built or Specialty GCP Clinical Systems

Specialty systems, such as electronic diaries, study monitoring systems, and remote data entry systems, are often developed or extensively modified in-house at trial sponsor companies. Custom spreadsheets and standard statistical macros are also frequently developed and may be used for more than one study or protocol in a particular therapeutic area. All such special software needs to be examined for its place on the matrix as GCP or non-GCP and then quality assured or validated accordingly.

Step 3: Identify Protocol-Specific Systems

A limitless variety of computerized systems and data devices can be used by protocols in today's clinical research environment. It is the responsibility of the trial sponsor's organization to identify all types of GCP electronic activity and e-data expected to be used during the conduct of prescribed clinical studies. One way to do this is to split the protocol systems planning between two groups:

- Have developers of the Medical Monitoring Plan study the protocol to identify GCP data systems used for diagnostic activities, for delivery or control of therapy, or for measurement of subject response to study therapy, and any other types of systems used to handle source data for CRFs at investigator sites.

- Have developers of the Data Management Plan study the protocol to determine GCP data system activities at CRO, laboratory, and sponsor sites, including network requirements among the three and with investigator sites.

Figure 11.3 shows typical types of computer systems used in a clinical study. All of the systems shown in the left-hand column of Figure 11.3 produce various types of raw data. The raw data may be in paper form that is later keyed into a system, or it may be collected as e-data from the point of generation. At some point, all study data becomes e-data and has to be processed, verified, reported, and archived. Establishing and managing electronic archives is a rather new concept for many third party providers of GCP e-data.

The types of computerized systems used by the protocol include both general and specialty systems. Remote data entry (RDE) systems usually require customized e-CRFs per study and can include components located at trial sponsor, CRO, and investigator sites. Special data transfer programs are often written for uploading study data from central laboratories and CROs, even when e-CRFs and RDE are not being used. An international protocol may require a software application such as a patient scheduler that converts a subject's height, weight, and other factors into

Figure 11.3. Protocol e-data systems planning

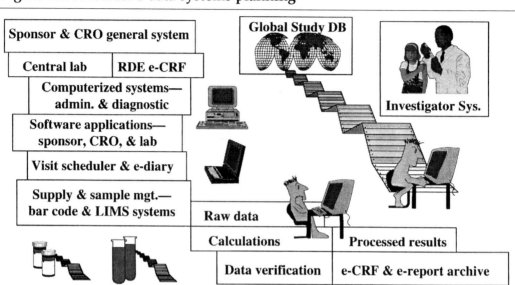

metric and nonmetric units and schedules visits according to the individual's response to therapy as defined by certain laboratory results.

Investigator sites can have a wide variety of GCP data systems that perform administrative, diagnostic, and treatment activities in studies. Sometimes, raw data is collected from monitoring systems that the subject wears. Other times, it may come from a medical device inside the patient such as a pacemaker, or a response measuring instrument may be used with which the subject interacts in the investigator's office. Some physicians write their observations on laptops.

Conducting studies around the world poses special problems for reconciling different company database definitions and for ensuring comparable medical evaluations and measurements by different investigators and their respective systems. Networking concerns for transmission speeds, data protection, and technology fit also arise. Such issues need to be examined and resolved before studies begin, so that clean data will be collected in a secure, timely fashion, and analysis of results across multiple sites will be valid. Clinical project schedules must include time for resolution of technology issues.

Step 4: Prepare e-Quality Action Sections for Medical Monitoring and Data Management Plans

Having identified GCP data systems, it is important to decide how to quality assure those systems and to include a section in the Medical Monitoring and Data Management Plans for actions to be taken in support of e-data and e-system quality (e-Quality/e-Q).

Medical Monitoring Action Plan

One practical way for a Monitoring Action Plan to reach investigator sites with e-Q concepts is by discussing them in the investigator's brochure with an emphasis on the e-data needs of the specific protocol. This topic should also be presented in training at investigator meetings. The trial sponsor's CRAs need to be trained in the e-Q needs of the protocol, in the messages of e-Q in the brochure, and in how to qualify and support a site in its ability to meet the critical e-data and technology needs of the study.

Data Management Action Plan

The Data Management Action Plan is likely to be far more detailed for e-Q than the medical monitoring one because it looks at the data needs of trial sponsor general systems as well as CRO, laboratory, and communications systems. This plan develops the protocol matrix of systems (Figure 11.2) and then decides what validation actions to take per system. It develops an e-Data Quality Plan (see Step Five) and trains CRAs in using the e-Data Quality (EDQ) Checklist. This plan includes collaboration activities with the IT department for *validation package* activities required by protocol-specific and general GCP systems.

Step 5: Develop an Electronic Data Quality Plan (EDQ Plan) for the Protocol

An Electronic Data Quality Plan (EDQ Plan) is a document which describes the strategy of a trial sponsor for addressing GCP compliance of e-data and e-system practices on a per study basis. It identifies those system activities that control therapy or handle SEQ data and are subject to validation compliance and audit and inspection activities.

To fully address the issue of e-data integrity, there are six categories of system activities to be considered. A specific trial protocol may have none, one, or many systems and applications to be considered among the following data handling categories:

1. *Data capture*—from a laboratory or medical instrument, a medical or therapeutic device, an electronic patient diary, an electrophysiology apparatus, or a pharmacy dispensing unit

2. *Data transformation*—calculation of raw data to an endpoint, conversion of raw data to graphical output, or statistical analysis of data

3. *Data transfer*—to, from, and among database systems at trial sponsor, CRO, central laboratory, and investigator sites

4. *Data management*—entry, storage, retrieval, and processing of data in a local or remote database structure

5. *Software development*—to customize spreadsheets, applications, and database structures for the requirements of a specific protocol

6. *Configuration management*—to apply GCP practices to all strategic systems used in items 1–5 above

The easiest way to build an EDQ Plan is for the Data Management Team to consider the CRF data elements from the view of an investigator's site, a CRO contractor, or a central laboratory, and then to consider the internal trial sponsor handling of CRF e-data. For each different view, an EDQ

Plan Checklist can then be designed to reflect the six e-data system concerns, plus other critical GCP issues. Such checklists can then be used as practical tools and guidance for CRAs and auditors who will be qualifying and monitoring sites involved in the studies.

One format for an EDQ Plan Checklist is shown in Figure 11.4 and examples of possible items have been given in italics. In the interests of space, this master checklist has example items for CRO, laboratory, and investigator sites all together, but for high technology protocols, it may be simpler to use separate checklists. A separate checklist should be made for trial sponsor systems to help data managers and the IT Department plan ahead for structuring databases and defining network guidance for expected data transfers from third parties. Early definition of database and network requirements makes it easier to include such requirements in supplier and site contracts, so that expectations are clear on both sides and the potential for data corruption or data loss is limited.

Step 6: Develop Practical Field Action Guidelines

The EDQ Plan Checklists can be used as a basis for developing field guidelines for CRAs and auditors to use pre-, during, and post-study. Field e-Quality Guidelines should help them to

- review a site's e-data and GCP systems capability for protocol-specific e-issues,
- identify sources of e-raw data,
- identify sources for e-CRFs and CRF e-data,
- monitor the integrity of GCP e-data at sites during studies, and
- plan a strategy for defending e-data integrity in post-trial inspections.

One way to provide guidance is by preparing sets of study questions that can be used by field personnel as direction for their own analysis or as prompts for interview

210   The Survive and Thrive Guide to Computer Validation

Figure 11.4. Electronic Data Quality (EDQ) Plan Checklist

EDQ Plan Checklist for clinical study: ID- _____

Trial sponsor representative:

_____

(Name)   (Title)   (Date)

Site representative: (CRO, central laboratory, investigator)

_____

(Name)   (Title)   (Date)

1. **Systems to be used at this site for electronic data capture in this protocol include the following:** (laboratory/medical instrumentation, medical/therapeutic device, patient diary, electrophysiology apparatus, pharmacy dispensing system, etc.)

List of data capture system(s)	Type(s) of data to be captured
a. *Patient diary*	a. *Pain and depression levels*
b. *Lab systems and LIMS*	b. *Blood drug levels*
c. *SAS workstation*	c. *Randomization codes*
d.	d.

2. **Electronic data calculations to be performed at this site for safety and efficacy data in this protocol include the following:** (formula to derive an endpoint value or next therapy dosage or transformation of instrument signals to graphical output, etc.)

Application software list	Type of calculation
a. *Dosage spreadsheet*	a. *Dosage based on blood levels*
b.	b.
c.	c.

3. **The transfer of electronic data to a local site database system or a remote sponsor system by this site in this protocol includes the following:** (Transfer methods could include phone modem, direct network link, diskette, tape, CD-ROM)

Type and source of electronic data	Transfer method	Data destination
a. *Lab results/LIMS system*	a. *modem*	a. *Sponsor's DB*
b. *Subject listings/CRO's SAS™*	b. *tape*	b. *Sponsor's DB*
c. *Subject's diary/diary device*	c. *diskette*	c. *Sponsor's DB*

Continued on next page.

Clinical Research Systems   **211**

Continued from previous page.

4. **Special data management issues for this protocol include the following:** (database structure requirements for special fields, audit trails, specific subsets of site information, etc.)

    a. Transferred data must be in sponsor-specified format as per contract document #478.

    b.

    c.

5. **Software development required for this protocol includes the following:** (to customize spreadsheets, applications, or database systems for the specific requirements of a protocol)

Software changes required	Party responsible
a. LIMS data subsets to fit sponsor's database structure	Lab staff
b. *SAS™ data sets to sponsor's format*	*Site/CRO contact*
c. *EXCEL™ spreadsheet written and tested*	*Sponsor and site*
d.	

6. **Configuration management for site systems used in data handling in this protocol will be administered as follows:** (SOPs, logbooks, *validation packages*, Systems QA Plan, etc.)

List of site system(s)	Site validation reference
a. *LIMS*	a. *Validation package and site SQAP*
b. *Subject diary device*	b. *Sponsor's validation package*
c. *SAS™ Workstation*	c. *Workstation Logbook and SOP*
d. *EXCEL™ dosage spreadsheet*	d. *Site's Testing Log*
e.	e.

7. **Authorization for making edits to electronic data in this protocol will be managed as follows:** (As per SOP, logbook, etc.)

    As per site SOP 98-25: Data change control authorization

Continued on next page.

212   The Survive and Thrive Guide to Computer Validation

Continued from previous page.

---

8.   **Responsibility for computerized systems delivered by the sponsor to the site for use in this trial are described below:**

System(s) Delivered	Validation package(s)	User SOPs
a. *Subject Diaries*	a. *Sponsor developed*	a. *Sponsor written*
b. *Dosage spreadsheet*	b. *Site's Testing Logbook*	b. *Site written*
c.	c.	c.

---

discussions with sites. Example study/interview questions for the six e-data integrity factors are given below:

1. *Electronic data capture:*
   - How is captured data to be monitored?
   - Are site personnel trained for the capture technology?
   - Is technology a part of the protocol plan?
   - How is GCP compliance maintained?
   - Can site personnel and the technology supplier support GCP and protocol needs?

2. *Computerized data calculation:*
   - How is the calculation documented?
   - Who wrote and tested the calculation program? Who fixes it?
   - Has a second method of calculation provided the same answers?
   - How is change control to be recorded for the calculation program and for calculated data?
   - How are users trained for it?

3. *Electronic data transfer:*
   - How is data to be moved between systems? By modem, fax, tape, diskette?

Clinical Research Systems   213

- What checks are made to ensure receipt of all data sent? Who resolves any problems?

- Are database systems compatible between systems? Do data fields, data types, and coded definitions match exactly?

4. *Data management:*

- Who is authorized to enter, edit, and retrieve data?

- How are audit, edit, and data trails kept?

- Is data modified to a new format prior to being transferred to the trial sponsor? How is this checked?

- How are edits to e-CRFs managed?

- What is the data backup and recovery process?

- How are missing values handled?

5. *Software development:*

- Does study protocol or site use require any special software, calculation, formula, or graphic?

- Does site equipment require modification of trial sponsor's software? If so, who does what to effect the changes?

- Is site e-data output compatible with trial sponsor's system?

- How is software documented, tested, fixed?

- How is change control maintained?

6. *Configuration management:*

- How are platform systems, software applications, and e-data to be monitored?

- Are records kept for service, backup, problem tracking, and repair activities?

- Who is responsible for system care and the backup of data?

- How is training provided for system and e-data users?

214 The Survive and Thrive Guide to Computer Validation

- What SOPs exist for security, testing, and disaster recovery of systems?

Another way for field guidelines to look at EDQ is by assessing system reliability factors for computer hardware and automated instrumentation and medical devices. Figure 11.5 gives a list of key reliability factors for regulated systems in general and GCP systems at any site.

III. Conclusion

Identify GCP Study Systems and Plan a Pragmatic Approach

Given the variety of computerized systems used in the practice of medicine today and the large amount of e-data produced in clinical trials, it is important to define system and e-data validation candidates in a simple way. The protocol matrix does this by identifying all systems based upon two factors:

Figure 11.5. Reliability factors for regulated systems

GCP systems and automated devices should

- be located in a clean, appropriate environment (temperature, humidity, dust)
- be installed and calibrated for use as per supplier's specifications
- be tested and checked for working limits with testing records kept
- be operated to written instructions (SOPs) after suitable training and with appropriate security controls
- be tested periodically for quality control of continued operation to expected standard
- be serviced and maintained at regular intervals with records kept
- have backup procedures for hardware, software, data, and communications
- have alternative arrangements prepared for disaster recovery from flood, fire, theft, and other hazards

1. Being trial sponsor owned or nonsponsor owned

2. Their handling of GCP data to make them GCP or non-GCP data systems

In the first case, standard system *validation packages* are developed by the trial sponsor's organization in usual fashion. In the second case, system *validation packages* are the responsibility of nonsponsor organizations (CRO, laboratory, Investigator) and the trial sponsor uses contract terms, site reviews, and audits to ensure the compliance of GCP e-data and systems.

Various regulatory directives such as the ICH GCP and the ICH Draft Guideline on Statistical Principles for Clinical Trials have common themes for protecting the integrity of electronic raw data and derived data in clinical studies. Validation of computerized systems is recognized as a necessary activity to ensure the integrity of GCP data. The system validation practices of Chapters 1–9 can be applied in a straightforward fashion to trial sponsor systems in order to meet such directives.

12. Manufacturing Systems

I. System Sponsor's Summary

Manufacturing today is filled with various types of computerized systems and embedded automation devices to the point where downtime for computers means downtime for production. This places a business imperative on having reliable systems that perform as intended. The business imperative is parallel to and supportive of regulatory demands for management control, data integrity, system reliability, and auditable quality of GMP systems. Given that financial, human, and system resources are always finite and must be carefully deployed, *sponsors* of manufacturing systems need to establish a definition for GMP systems at their facility and give a rationale for prioritizing validation resources to address compliance. Figure 12.1 gives a commonly used set of definitions for identifying GMP systems.

GMP Status and Validation Priority

Experience has shown that companies put the safety of personnel first on the priority list along with product safety. The concept of product safety includes both the physical safety of the product during manufacturing and distribution and the product as safe for use by the ultimate consumer. In this framework, GMP status and *first validation priority* would go to computerized systems whose malfunction would cause

- safety problems for personnel operating it,
- safety problems for the product itself,

The Survive and Thrive Guide to Computer Validation

Figure 12.1. Concept definitions—GMP systems

GMP computerized systems:

1. **Control the quality of product** during its development, testing, manufacturing and handling.

2. **Handle data used to prove** the **safety, efficacy** and **quality** of product and formulation

3. **Have a direct impact on** the **safety of personnel** during a system malfunction.

- safety problems for the consumers of the product, or

- loss or corruption of safety data about the product.

GMP status and *second validation priority* would go to systems controlling efficacy characteristics of the product and handling data about the efficacy of the product, such as the amount of active therapeutic ingredient per unit of product or the potency of a batch over time. GMP status and *third validation priority* would go to systems controlling other quality characteristics of the product and handling other quality data about the product or manufacturing process, such as level of cleanliness of air, quality of water, sterility of containers, clarity of liquid, uniformity of color and shape, thoroughness of cleaning between batches, processing temperatures, and mixing times.

Once the GMP systems have been identified and prioritized, the question arises, "How much is enough for validation work?" The first answer is that perfection is not required, but responsible action is. The EU Guide to GMP Annex 11 on computerized systems gives a very simple definition of the need as shown in Figure 12.2.

Such a definition is also in agreement with basic management principles that would probably expect even more ROI from computerized systems and production automation.

Most manufacturing operations expect to improve on the quality of product and process with investments in computerized systems and automation and not just stay the same as previous levels of manual operation.

The application of computer validation practices to develop standard packages for strategic GMP systems is the surest way to achieve both regulatory and business goals for product and process quality and quality assurance. The EU GMP Annex 11 also provides a concise statement of computer validation practices required for compliance (Figure 12.3). As discussed in Chapter 8, the validation practices described in the 19 paragraphs of Annex 11 are also endorsed by all of the other international regulations that focus on Good Practice compliance of computer systems.

II. System Owner and System Team Discussion

It is important to have a strategy for looking at computer systems in manufacturing. After establishing the GMP status and priority of facility-wide systems such as MRP

Figure 12.2 What's the basic concern?

EU GMP Guide Annex 11: Computerized Systems
Principle:
Product quality and quality assurance should not decrease when a computerized system replaces a manual operation.

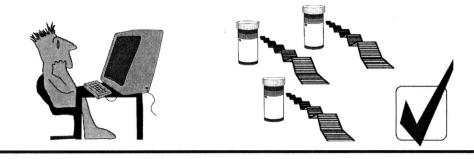

220 The Survive and Thrive Guide to Computer Validation

Figure 12.3. EU GMP Annex 11 requirements

Management control	System reliability
• Principle—product quality	• Software quality assurance (5)
• Personnel (1)	• Testing (7)
• Validation/life cycle management (2)	• Control of change (11)
• System environment (3)	• Alternative arrangements (15)
• Supplier contracts (18)	• Recovery procedures (16)
• Release security (19)	
Data integrity	**Auditable quality**
• Built-in entry & processing checks (6)	• System description (4)
• System security (8)	• Audit trail—entry & edits (10)
• Verification of critical data (9)	• Paper copies—data audits (12)
• Data integrity (13)	• Error tracking (17)
• Data backup (14)	

and environment control heating, ventilation, and air conditioning (HVAC) systems, it can be confusing for *system owners* and *system teams* to sort a work path through the variety of configurations used in the production process. There are so many different types of systems from programmable logic controllers (PLCs) inside equipment to distributed control systems (DCSs), software control and data acquisition systems (SCADAs), networked PCs, and laboratory systems.

How can a manufacturer use business-based logic to design a project that addresses computer validation in a realistic way? Some of the most common business reasons to design computer validation projects for GMP systems include the following:

- Construction of a plant expansion or new facility to include automated GMP systems

- Configuration of an automated production line for a newly approved GMP product

- Introduction of regulated product into previously non-GMP production facilities

- Purchase of a new facility-wide GMP system such as MRP, integrated production control, or electronic signatures for batch records

Experience has shown that one practical approach to working with GMP systems validation is that given in the eight-step program that follows.

Step 1: Conduct a Walk-Through of the Facility or New Product Life Cycle

When starting a new program of system validation, conduct a walk-through and Gap Analysis exercise to identify all GMP systems for the area of interest. The single system walk-through process discussed in Chapter 6 can be adapted to cover multiple systems at a higher level in order to inventory, classify (GMP/non-GMP), and prioritize (SEQ) them for further validation efforts. The walk-through could be for the whole manufacturing site or for a particular facility, department, or production line on the site (Figure 12.4).

Various configurations of large and small systems and applications can be observed throughout a site. If a C.V. Policy has been established for the site, there may be one or more SQAPs available to help the team review systems and their level of compliance. Usually, there will be a Master Plan for the site that identifies any expected major construction changes, any major new systems to be installed, and the types of products to be manufactured there. Process execution systems, such as mixing, filling, labeling, and checking systems, can vary from a single embedded chip or PLC to a large DCS or SCADA system.

The answer to the question, "What is computerized?" can be, "Almost everything!" When a computerized system has been identified, the next walk-through question is, "Where is the system located and is the environment suitable for the system?" Other questions follow:

Figure 12.4. GMP systems at a manufacturing site

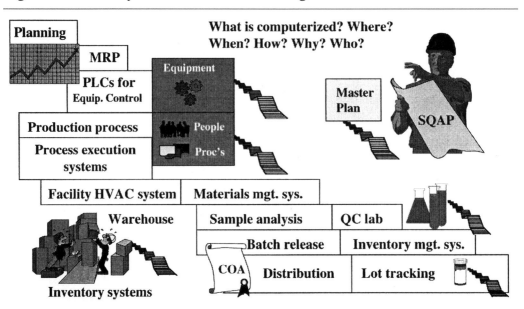

- *Who* is responsible for this system? The system sponsor? The system owner?
- *What* is the intended purpose of this system? Is it GMP relevant?
- *Where* are the records for testing and operating the system? For training users?
- *When* was the system installed, and when was it last maintained?
- *Why* would failure of this system have an impact on SEQ issues for GMP product, data, or personnel?
- *How* is the system controlled for security and operation, and is there documentation to support the control?

Alternatively, a walk-through could review computerized systems used for producing a new or current product by following the life cycle of that particular product in detail from the initial order to build it through production to its Certificate of Analysis (COA) and release for distribution off the warehouse loading dock. A regulated product is usually required to have a Master Validation Plan developed to ensure fully documented operations for the quality of the process used to make it. As the process has become more and more electronic, a new focus on documented quality for the computerized part of the process has become of regulatory concern. Since computer validation tends to be the "forgotten stepchild" in most product Master Validation Plans, a separate focus is needed for it and a Walk-Through Report can provide this.

Step 2: Develop a C.V. Policy Statement and an SQAP

The site should have a Computer Validation Policy Statement that is approved and signed by local management. The corporate C.V. Policy can be used with a cover memo that gives the supporting views and commitment of local management to policy practices. A C.V. Policy Statement can then be written to establish a local executive review group to monitor site compliance to the C.V. Policy. If no corporate policy exists, the site can develop its own as per Chapter 7.

With the local C.V. Policy Statement and/or C.V. Policy in place, a Site Team of *system owners* can develop an SQAP to translate the C.V. Policy into what it means for GMP systems and local practice at the site. As discussed in Chapter 6, the SQAP would give guidance to all personnel involved in system validation work. It would define for the site the validation roles and responsibilities for the following:

- System management (*sponsors* and *owners*)
- GMP quality assurance (QA)
- System quality control (SQC)
- Operations (users)
- Plant engineering and maintenance (PLC and HVAC suppliers)
- The IT Department (platform systems, infrastructure, and software supplier)

224 The Survive and Thrive Guide to Computer Validation

- Outside contractors (DCS, SCADA, and MRP suppliers)

- Subcontractors for product production (contract manufacturers)

An addendum to the SQAP should describe a Way Forward Business Plan with a prioritized approach to systems validation for the current fiscal year and the next fiscal year. The Way Forward Plan should reference specific project support approved by management, such as a list (by job title, not name) of *system sponsors* and *owners* for the prioritized systems, and budget line items for validation resources for the current year's work. Such a business plan commitment shows due diligence on the part of management for implementation of the SQAP.

Step 3: Standard Operating Procedures

As per Chapter 8, GMP regulations in the United States (Figure 8.5) and Japan (Figure 8.12) give topics to be covered by SOP for manufacturing systems. For laboratory systems, the site can refer to the OECD GLP list of SOPs (Figure 4.11) and Chapter 10 with the GALP list of system SOPs (Figure 10.3). There is plenty of guidance available, and the major concern is not to overdo SOP writing. It is important to keep directions as simple and understandable as possible with no confusing duplication of information sources.

The use of three levels of SOP described in the documentation model of Chapter 7 is designed specifically to reduce duplication of effort (Figure 12.5). The site should have only one general SOP for how to manage GMP system suppliers and not separate ones for different departments and systems. There should be only one general site SOP for how to create, handle, and archive system validation documentation. There should be only one general site SOP for how to respond to system audits and inspections, and perhaps it is just a systems section in an SOP that already covers audit and inspection response for everything else at the site.

Local SOPs might cover testing practices for all GMP systems in sterile environments, software engineering practices for writing PLC logic, data center practices for configuration management of GMP platform systems, or laboratory practices for the calibration and backup of multiple chromatography data systems of a particular type. The more that common practices can be agreed and incorporated into local department or area SOPs, the less work is left for writing SOPs at the system standard *validation package* level. Whenever the system *validation package* can reference local or general SOPs in its Validation Plan or Test Plan, there is no need to duplicate the information in the *validation package*. In addition, it becomes an inspector-friendly situation with SOPs providing a consistent approach across multiple systems showing management control for implementing computer validation practices.

System and user SOPs would then only be used for the specific procedures required that are unique to the single system. It may even be that for some systems, written tech-

Figure 12.5. Site Computer Validation documentation model

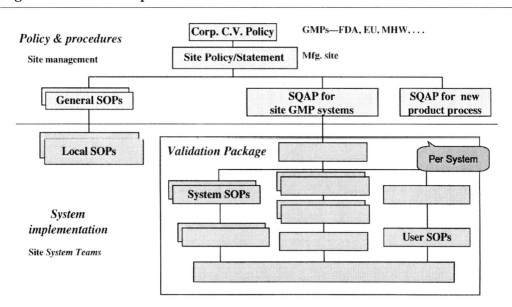

The Survive and Thrive Guide to Computer Validation

nical instructions can be used instead of the more formal SOP process when local and general SOPs cover most of the system requirements.

Step 4: Assign System Teams and Develop Standard Validation Packages

A walk-through list of GMP systems can be prioritized according to the relevant SQAP guidelines and have *system owners* and *system teams* assigned to develop standard *validation packages* for them as per Chapters 3–5. The EU GMP Guide Annex 11 recommends essentially the same life cycle approach as the one described in Chapter 2 and also discusses sizing the validation effort to fit the system situation.[1]

Validation
2. The extent of validation necessary will depend on a number of factors including the use to which the system is to be put, whether the validation is to be prospective or retrospective, and whether or not novel elements are incorporated. Validation should be considered as part of the complete life cycle of a computer system. This life cycle includes the stages of planning, specification, programming, testing, commissioning, documentation, operation, monitoring, and modifying.

The mention of "novel elements" refers to any customized code being developed for the configuration at an particular site and includes such items as "bug fixes" and other modifications or enhancements of software and hardware such as in PLCs. A very important consideration for both Validation Plans and Test Plans is the system practice for problem resolution that has change control procedures for fixes and enhancements to the system that include criteria for testing the system *after* installation of the "novel element" and *prior to* resuming normal operation.

---

1. Guide to Good Manufacturing Practice for Medicinal Products—Annex 11: Computerized Systems, *The Rules Governing Medicinal Products in the European Union*, Volume IV (Office for Official Publications of the European Communities, Luxemburg, January 1992), p. 139.

In the fast-paced manufacturing environment, there is often intense pressure to "just fix it and do the testing later," that usually translates into running an out-of-validation system and frequently forgotten testing. In the luckiest of situations, such an untested "quick fix" allows operations to continue smoothly. Often, however, such a quick fix results in unexpected side effects within the system that result in problems in other areas of the computerized process. With luck, these side-effect problems may easily be seen, but they can also become visible only after one or more batches of substandard (out-of-specification) product have been made. Either way, waste of product and rework becomes an expense that exceeds the cost of performing the fix properly the first time with appropriate testing to keep the system in a reliable and validated state.

Another area for careful consideration is that of documentation for "novel elements." A bug fix documentation process should be established that records sufficient detail to support the continued maintenance activities of the system, but does not overburden support personnel in getting the job done in a reasonable time. This could be accomplished with a local department SOP to define the essential information requirements in a format that is convenient to use and reflects the agreed practice among professionals in the department who have to produce the fixes.

Step 5: Train All Site Personnel to GMP System Validation Concepts

It is important that all site personnel come to realize that maintaining GMP for computerized systems is just as important and just as much a part of their jobs as working to GMP for making product. In fact it is all part of the *same* job. People tend to have one of several responses to computerized systems. They take them for granted and think of them as glorified typewriters or calculators, they consider them to be "magic boxes" that can do no wrong, they think of them as devices for playing video games, or they think that computers are too complicated and are afraid of them. None of these responses is healthy in a GMP environment.

The goal of GMP computer validation training for site personnel should be to teach people how to support the quality assurance of electronic data and systems as a normal part of their work activities. A person should know what GMP computerized systems they use on their job, and should seek training for how to use them in compliance to GMP. The importance of calibration, testing, maintenance, and documentation of GMP computer systems is similar to other equipment requirements under GMP that people already understand and practice.

Training materials in system *validation packages* should reflect any parallels to production validation efforts in order to make it easier for users on all shifts to understand, accept, and implement system SOPs appropriately in their work. Using or adapting practices and formats already established at the site for logbook entries and other types of recordkeeping can help people accept the documentation practices for the operation and maintenance activities required for GMP systems. The application of GMP to computerized systems then has a familiar look and feel for users.

Step 6: Take a Product Life Cycle Approach to Large and Legacy Systems

Sometimes it is difficult to know where to start a validation focus for very large and complex systems, such as integrated MRP and warehousing systems, or for automation that has been in operation for some time (legacy systems). For such systems, the GMP status decision and the SEQ prioritization can be made from a logical point of view if the *system team* studies how manufacturing a particular product at the site requires the use of such systems.

The *system team* conducts a physical walk-through tour of the whole life cycle of the product. The tour begins with receipt on site of an order to build Product "X" and then proceeds through the whole production process out to release and distribution of a lot of Product "X" from the warehouse shipping dock (Figure 12.6). This process can also be

Figure 12.6. GMP systems—product "X" view

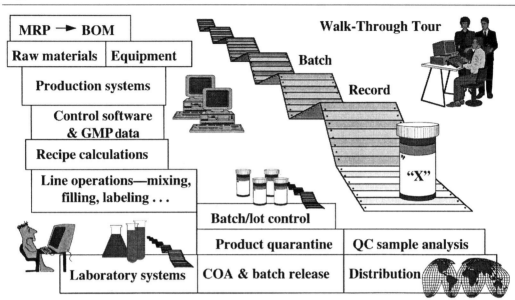

helpful in preparing for a pre-approval inspection of the site for a New Drug Application (NDA).

The walk-through tour maps three paths through the Product "X" view of GMP systems at the site. The first path maps the physical activities required to make Product "X." The second path identifies all points of electronic data handling or electronic process control associated with the physical activity. The third path identifies the system performing each activity and evaluates the GMP status and SEQ priority of the system (Figure 12.7). One way to make the evaluation is to answer the following questions: "What are the consequences of a system failure during this activity?" and "In what way(s) could the system fail at this point?"

This process can be very instructive in the case of legacy systems whose identity and documentation may have become obscure and out-of-date over time. It can also uncover undocumented new uses of a system that have been developed by operators to meet special work situations. In

230   The Survive and Thrive Guide to Computer Validation

Figure 12.7. Describing GMP Systems for Product "X"

Perform a walk-through of the site life cycle for Product "X" and note the following:

Site activity	Electronic points	System ID—GMP/SEQ status
1. Process requisition	1. Key in order form	1. Admin.—non-GMP
2. Generate Bill of Materials (BOM)	2. Query MRP system to check raw materials	2. Materials Mgt.—GMP/SEQ function in MRP

the Walk-Through Report, the systems identified can be prioritized for validation work with safety impact first, efficacy impact second, and other quality systems third. The application of SEQ analysis can be used through numerous levels of a process or a system to help prioritize efforts within a large system or validation project.

Step 7: Plan for Electronic Records Retention and Electronic Signature Use

The great number of signed records required during the production of regulated product has led to a strong interest in the use of electronic records and electronic signatures to reduce the need for paper records. These become particularly important in sterile manufacturing areas where paper is not allowed. As discussed in Chapter 8, the U.S. FDA has published its Final Rule on e-records and e-signatures so that guidelines do exist to support the validation and use of these systems (Figure 12.8).[2]

---

2. 21 CFR Part 11—Electronic Records; Electronic Signatures; Final Rule. *Federal Register.* Thursday, March 20,1997, p. 13465.

Figure 12.8. FDA Final Rule: e-records and e-signature

Scope:

... systems to create, modify, maintain, or transmit electronic records shall employ *procedures and controls designed to ensure the authenticity, integrity, and,* when appropriate, *the confidentiality of electronic records,* and to ensure that the *signer cannot readily reject* the signed record as not genuine.

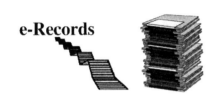
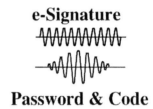

For all types of e-record systems, the FDA set forth a list of control practices that echoes all of the common computer validation themes, while placing its focus on systems for e-records and e-signatures (refer to Figure 9.3). It is important to note that document encryption is not one of the normal controls recommended. It is only when GMP records reside on open systems with access controlled by parties having no GMP responsibility that the rule says document encryption may be used "as necessary" to ensure e-record authenticity, integrity, and confidentiality.

When site functions decide to use electronic signatures, they must establish and implement a general SOP defining how to verify the identity of an individual prior to assignment of an e-signature and have that individual certify in writing that their e-signature is the legally binding equivalent of their traditional handwritten signature.

Electronic signatures that are not based on biometrics must employ at least two distinct identification components, such as an identification code and a password. If an e-signature must be executed when the genuine owner is unavailable, the system must require the collaboration of two or more individuals to execute it. The use of e-signatures with e-records brings out a concern about the ability to "cut and paste" a signature to create a false record. This concern is addressed in Section 11.70 of the Final Rule (Figure 12.9).[3]

Step 8: Prepare for Audits and Inspections

It is important that all site personnel understand their role for any audit or inspection of the systems they use. Second- and third-shift personnel should also be trained in how to respond to an audit and inspection situation. There should be a designated response team of two or more individuals on each shift who are prepared to answer all the questions in the general checklist of Figure 9.6 for strategic GMP systems used on that shift. The answers to these questions can also be used as part of the training program for new system users.

Figure 12.9. FDA Final Rule: Section 11.70

Signature/record linking:

Electronic signatures and handwritten signatures executed to e-records shall be linked to their respective e-records to ensure that *the signatures cannot be excised, copied, or otherwise transferred to falsify an e-record by ordinary means.*

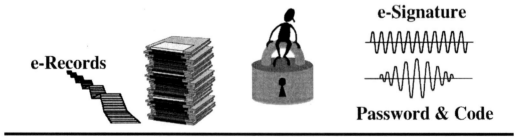

---

3. 21 CFR 11, p. 13466.

A part of general GMP training for all personnel should include guidance on how to participate in reviews, audits, and inspections. The concepts of direct, truthful answers to direct questions and the non volunteering of "war stories" about problem fixes or repeating gossip about system situations in other areas need to be communicated to all individuals on all shifts. Every system user on every shift should be able to locate SOPs and logbooks associated with their use of the system. They should also be able to demonstrate their use of the system in a way that is compliant with system documentation and should keep their training records updated for training on the systems they operate. On a periodic basis, *system owners* would be wise to spot-check users for their audit preparedness on these items.

III. Conclusion

Product "X" Life Cycle Approach and SEQ Priority

The complexity of integrated systems and automated production in manufacturing today presents site management with a serious challenge for sorting out a practical approach to computer validation. Performing a walk-through of systems used in the site life cycle for making a specific product (Product "X") can help *system teams* decide GMP status and SEQ priority for the systems used in making that product. The same process can also work at a deeper level to prioritize (SEQ) validation effort for modules of a system based on how it performs in the production of the chosen product.

Structuring a supportive environment for computer validation with Policy, SQAP, standard *validation packages,* and SOPs puts computer validation on a par with other process validation as being part of normal GMP work activity. Clear guidance for prioritizing systems and a convenient framework of standard documents for implementing compliance makes the job easier to accomplish.

13. GMP References (EU and Japan), Electronic Records and Electronic Signatures (US)

Introduction—Document Contacts

In this chapter are excerpts from various regulations and guidelines for Good Manufacturing Practice in the pharmaceutical and biopharmaceutical industries. Experience has shown that these documents are very useful to *system teams* performing the practical work of computer validation. Original copies of these documents may be obtained through their regulatory sources. The FDA on-line service can actually download documents directly to the requester's computer.

European Union (EU)

All regulatory documents are available through

> Office for Official Publications of the European Communities
> 2 rue Mercier
> L-2985 LUXEMBURG

Ministry of Health and Welfare (MHW) Japan

English translations of MHW regulatory documents are available from

> Yakuji Nippo, Ltd.
> 1, Kanda Isumicho, Chiyoda-ku,
> Tokyo, 101 JAPAN
> Tel:+81-3-3862-2141
> Fax: +81-3-5621-8757

236   The Survive and Thrive Guide to Computer Validation

U.S. Food and Drug Administration (FDA)

All U.S. and ICH regulatory documents are available through the FDA's Internet home page at

http://www.fda.gov

GMP References, Electronic Records and Signatures 237

EU GMP GUIDE—Annex 11 and Excerpts of Chapters 4 and 7

Source: The Rules Governing Medicinal Products in the European Union, Volume IV, Good Manufacturing Practice for Medicinal Products in the European Union, III/5061/96, January 1992. European Commission Directorate-General III—Industry. Pages 33–34, 59–61, 139–142.

Annex 11—Pages 139–142
11. Computerized Systems

Principle

The introduction of computerized systems into systems of manufacturing, including storage, distribution and quality control does not alter the need to observe the relevant principles given elsewhere in the Guide. Where a computerized system replaces a manual operation, there should be no resultant decrease in product quality and quality assurance. Consideration should be given to the risk of losing aspects of the previous system which could result form reducing the involvement of operators.

Personnel

1.   It is essential that there is the closest cooperation between key personnel and those involved with computer systems. Persons in responsible positions should have the appropriate training for the management and use of systems within their field of responsibility which utilize computers. This should include insuring that appropriate expertise is available and used to provide advice on aspects of design, validation, installation, and operation of computerized systems.

Validation

2.   The extent of validation necessary will depend on a number of factors including the use to which the system is to be put, whether the validation is to be prospective or retrospective and whether or not novel items are incorporated. Validation should be considered as part of the complete life cycle of a computer system. This cycle includes the stages of planning, specification, programming, testing, commissioning, documentation, operation, monitoring and modifying.

System

3.   Attention should be paid to the siting of equipment in suitable conditions where extraneous factors cannot interfere with the system.

238   The Survive and Thrive Guide to Computer Validation

4.   A written detailed description of the system should be produced (including diagrams as appropriate) and kept up to date. It should describe the principles, objectives, security measures and scope of the system and the main features of the way in which the computer is used and how it interacts with other systems and procedures.

5.   The software is a critical component of a computerized system. The user of such software should take all reasonable steps to ensure that it has been produced in accordance with a system of Quality Assurance.

6.   The system should include, where appropriate, built-in checks of the correct entry and processing of data.

7.   Before a system using a computer is brought into use, it should be thoroughly tested and confirmed as being capable of achieving the desired results. If a manual system is being replaced, the two should be run in parallel for a time, as a part of this testing and validation.

8.   Data should only be entered or amended by persons authorized to do so. Suitable methods of deterring unauthorized entry of data include the use of keys, passwords, personal codes and restricted access to computer terminals. There should be a defined procedure for the issue, cancellation, and alteration of authorization to enter and amend data, including the changing of personal passwords. Consideration should be given to systems allowing for recording of attempts to access by unauthorized persons.

9.   When critical data are being entered manually (for example, weight and batch number of an ingredient during dispensing), there should be an additional check on the accuracy of the record which is made. This check may be done by a second operator or by validated electronic means.

10.   The system should record the identity of operators entering or confirming critical data. Authority to amend entered data should be restricted to nominated persons. Any alteration to an entry of critical data should be authorized and recorded with the reason for the change. Consideration should be given to building into the system the creation of a complete record of all entries and amendments (an "audit trail").

11.   Alterations to a system or to a computer program should only be made in accordance with a defined procedure which should include provision for validating, checking, approving, and implementing the change. Such an alteration should only be implemented with the agreement of the person responsible for the part of the system concerned, and the alteration should be recorded. Every significant modification should be validated.

12.   For quality auditing purposes, it should be possible to obtain clear printed copies of electronically stored data.

GMP References, Electronic Records and Signatures 239

13. Data should be secured by physical or electronic means against willful or accidental damage, in accordance with item 4.9 of the Guide. Stored data should be checked for accessibility, durability and accuracy. If changes are proposed to the computer equipment or its programs, the above-mentioned checks should be performed at a frequency appropriate for the storage medium being used.

14. Data should be protected by backing up at regular intervals. Backup data should be stored as long as necessary at a separate and secure location.

15. There should be available adequate alternative arrangements for systems which need to be operated in the event of a breakdown. The time required to bring the alternative arrangements into use should be related to the possible urgency of the need to use them. For example, information required to effect a recall must be available at short notice.

16. The procedures to be followed if the system fails or breaks down should be defined and validated. Any failures and remedial action taken should be recorded.

17. A procedure should be established to record and analyze errors and to enable corrective action to be taken.

18. When outside agencies are used to provide a computer service, there should be a formal agreement, including a clear statement of the responsibilities of that outside agency (see Chapter 7).

19. When the release of batches for sale or supply is carried out using a computerized system, the system should allow for only a Qualified Person to release the batches, and it should clearly identify and record the person releasing the batches.

EU GMP Guide Chapter 4
Documentation

Principle

Good documentation constitutes an essential part of the quality assurance system. Clearly written documentation prevents errors from spoken communication and permits tracing of batch history. Specifications, manufacturing formulae and instructions, procedures, and records must be free from errors and available in writing. The legibility of documents is of paramount importance.

General

(Items 4.1 and 4.2 are not applicable to computers.)

240 The Survive and Thrive Guide to Computer Validation

4.3 Documents should be approved, signed and dated by appropriate and authorized persons.

4.4 Documents should have unambiguous contents; title, nature and purpose should be clearly stated. They should be laid out in an orderly fashion and be easy to check. Reproduced documents should be clear and legible. The reproduction of working documents from master documents must not allow any error to be introduced through the reproduction process.

4.5 Documents should be regularly reviewed and kept up-to-date. When a document has been revised, systems should be operated to prevent inadvertent use of superseded documents.

4.6 Documents should not be handwritten; although, where documents require the entry of data, these entries may be made in clear, legible, indelible handwriting. Sufficient space should be provided for such entries.

4.7 Any alteration made to the entry on a document should be signed and dated; the alteration should permit the reading of the original information. Where appropriate, the reason for the alteration should be recorded.

4.8 The records should be made or completed at the time each action is taken and in such a way that all significant activities concerning the manufacture of medicinal products are traceable. They should be retained for at least one year after the expiry date of the finished product.

4.9 Data may be recorded by electronic data processing systems, photographic or other reliable means, but detailed procedures relating to the system in use should be available and the accuracy of the records should be checked. If documentation is handled by electronic data processing methods, only authorized persons should be able to enter or modify data in the computer, and there should be a record of changes and deletions; access should be restricted by passwords or other means, and the result of entry of critical data should be independently checked. Batch records electronically stored should be protected by backup transfer on magnetic tape, microfilm, paper, or other means. It is particularly important that the data are readily available throughout the period of retention.

EU GMP Guide Chapter 7
Contract Manufacture and Analysis

Principle

Contract manufacture and analysis must be correctly defined, agreed, and controlled in order to avoid misunderstandings which could result in a product or

GMP References, Electronic Records and Signatures   241

work of unsatisfactory quality. There must be a written contract between the Contract Giver and the Contract Acceptor which clearly establishes the duties of each party. The contract must clearly state the way in which the Qualified Person releasing each batch of product for sale exercises his full responsibility.

Note: This chapter deals with the responsibilities of manufacturers towards the Competent Authorities of the Member States with respect to the granting of marketing and manufacturing authorizations. It is not intended in any way to affect the respective liability of contract acceptors and contract givers to consumers; this is governed by other provisions of Community and national law.

General

7.1   There should be a written contract covering the manufacture and/or analysis arranged under contract and any technical arrangements made in connection with it.

7.2   All arrangements for contract manufacture and analysis including any proposed changes in technical or other arrangements should be in accordance with the marketing authorization for the product concerned.

The Contract Giver

7.3   The Contract Giver is responsible for assessing the competence of the Contract Acceptor to carry out successfully the work required and for ensuring by means of the contract that the principles and guidelines of GMP as interpreted in this Guide are followed.

7.4   The Contract Giver should provide the Contract Acceptor with all the information necessary to carry out the contracted operations correctly in accordance with the marketing authorization and any other legal requirements. The Contract Giver should ensure that the Contract Acceptor is fully aware of any problems associated with the product or the work which might pose a hazard to his premises, equipment, personnel, other materials or other products.

7.5   The Contract Giver should ensure that all processed products and materials delivered to him by the Contract Acceptor comply with their specifications or that the products have been released by a Qualified Person.

The Contract Acceptor

7.6   The Contract Acceptor must have adequate premises and equipment, knowledge and experience, and competent personnel to carry out satisfactorily the work ordered by the Contract Giver. Contract manufacture

242   The Survive and Thrive Guide to Computer Validation

may be undertaken only by a manufacturer who is the holder of a manufacturing authorization.

7.7   The Contract Acceptor should ensure that all products or materials delivered to him are suitable for their intended purpose.

7.8   The Contract Acceptor should not pass to a third party any of the work entrusted to him under the contract without the Contract Giver's prior evaluation and approval of the arrangements. Arrangements made between the Contract Acceptor and any third party should ensure that the manufacturing and analytical information is made available in the same way as between the original Contract Giver and Contract Acceptor.

7.9   The Contract Acceptor should refrain from any activity which may adversely affect the quality of the product manufactured and/or analyzed for the Contract Giver.

The Contract

7.10   A contract should be drawn up between the Contract Giver and the Contract Acceptor which specifies their respective responsibilities relating to the manufacture and control of the product. Technical aspects of the contract should be drawn up by competent persons suitably knowledgeable in pharmaceutical technology, analysis, and Good Manufacturing Practice. All arrangements for manufacture and analysis must be in accordance with the marketing authorization and agreed by both parties.

7.11   The contract should specify the way in which the Qualified Person releasing the batch for sale ensures that each batch has been manufactured and checked for compliance with the requirements of the Marketing Authorization.

7.12   The contract should describe clearly who is responsible for purchasing materials, testing and releasing materials, undertaking production and quality controls, including in-process controls, and who has responsibility for sampling and analysis. In the case of contract analysis, the contract should state whether or not the Contract Acceptor should take samples at the premises of the manufacturer.

7.13   Manufacturing, analytical, and distribution records, and reference samples should be kept by, or be available to, the Contract Giver. Any records relevant to assessing the quality of the product in the event of complaints or a suspected defect must be accessible and specified in the defect/recall procedures of the Contract Giver.

7.14   The contract should permit the Contract Giver to visit the facilities of the Contract Acceptor.

GMP References, Electronic Records and Signatures   243

7.15   In the case of contract analysis, the Contract Acceptor should understand that he is subject to inspection by the competent Authorities.

MHW—Japan—Guideline on Control of Computerized Systems in Drug Manufacturing

Part 1: Objectives

This guideline shall govern drug manufacturing plants where "Good Manufacturing Practices for Pharmaceutical Products (MHW Ordinance No. 31, 16 Aug. 1983)" and/or "Good Manufacturing Practices for Bulk Drug Substances (PAB Notification No. 598, 15 July 1988)" (hereafter referred to as Drug GMP and other regulations) is enforced. This guideline provides the guiding principles for the development and utilization of computer systems (hereinafter including all devices and equipment controlled by a computer) in process control, production control, quality control, etc. which ensures the appropriate implementation of Drug GMP and other regulations.

Part 2: Scope of Application

This guideline shall apply to the drug manufacturing plants governed by Drug GMP and other regulations where any of the following systems are introduced. However, systems with limited function that are operated simply by inputting parameters into a program fixed by the supplier of the hardware (including every device and equipment controlled by the computer) as general functions of the devices shall be exempted from this guideline.

1.   The system for manufacturing process control and management including that recording these data

2.   The system for production control such as storage and inventory of starting materials and final products including intermediates

3.   The system for documentation of manufacturing directions, testing protocols, or records

4.   The system for quality control and recording of these data

244   The Survive and Thrive Guide to Computer Validation

Part 3: Development of the System

3.1 System Designing

3.1.1 Key Personnel

A.   The manufacturer shall designate a manager and person/s in charge of each step of the system development ranging from "system engineering" (see 3.2) to "installation and operation" (see 3.5). The same person may also assume the responsibility for several steps of the system development.

B.   The manager shall specify individual duties of person/s in charge.

3.1.2 System Development Manual

The manufacturer shall document a system development manual which shall normally include:

A.   Procedures of system development.

B.   Documents to be prepared during each step of system development and the methods of maintaining these documents.

C.   Procedures for evaluation and approval of each step of system development.

D.   Procedures for amending or repeal of the system development manual.

3.1.3 Development Schedule

The manufacturer shall prepare a development schedule which in general shall describe the following:

A.   Objectives of the system development

B.   Time table of the system development

C.   Mobilization of staff

D.   Criteria for hardware selection

E.   Equipment arrangement for hardware installation

GMP References, Electronic Records and Signatures   245

3.2 System Engineering

3.2.1 The System Engineering Document

The manufacturer shall prepare a system engineering document which includes, in principle, the following:

A.   Composition of hardware

B.   Outline of system function

C.   Tabulation of input/output data

D.   File composition outline

E.   Countermeasures against system shutdown

F.   Security control function

G.   Title or name of the manager and person/s in charge

3.2.2 Approval of the System Engineering Document

The manager shall ensure that the above system engineering document be prepared in accordance with the provisions of the development manual.

3.3 Program Development

3.3.1 Preparation of Program Specification

The manager shall ensure that the person/s in charge prepare a program specification which includes, in principle, the following:

A.   Details of input/output data

B.   Details of data processing

C.   Title or name of the manager and person/s in charge

3.3.2 Evaluation of Program Specification and the Program

A.   The manager shall ensure that the program specification be established in conformity with the system engineering document.

B.   The manager shall ensure that the program is written according to the program specification.

246   The Survive and Thrive Guide to Computer Validation

3.3.3   Trial Test for the Program

A   The manager shall ensure that the person/s in charge prepare a trial test plan for the program, including test methods and evaluation criteria of the test results.

B.   The person/s in charge shall keep a record of the results of the program trial test in accordance with the provision of the trial test plan for the program.

C.   The manager shall evaluate the results of the program trial test and thereafter approve it.

3.4   *System Performance Test*

3.4.1   System Performance Test Plan

The Manager shall ensure that person/s in charge prepare a system performance test (this will confirm the performance of the system, such as storing the program and running satisfactorily in compliance with the design specification in the non-production condition) plan including the following items:

A.   Conditions of the system performance test (such as interface of hardware, program composition, etc.)

B.   Check items of the system performance test and test data used

C.   Method of the system performance test and evaluation of the test results

D.   Time table of the system performance test

E.   Job allocation during the system performance test

3.4.2   Implementation of the System Performance Test

A.   Person/s in charge shall conduct the system performance test and maintain test records (Including system problems observed during the test and corrective measures taken), according to the system performance test plan.

B.   The manager shall evaluate the test results and approve them thereafter. The evaluation criteria of the system performance test are, in principle, as follows:

    a.   Function—does it match the provisions of the system engineering document, etc.

    b.   Capability—assurance of the system response as designed in the system engineering document, etc.

GMP References, Electronic Records and Signatures 247

    c.   Reliability—does every function work satisfactorily, etc.

    d.   Operation—appropriateness of operation of terminal devices, etc.

3.5 Installation and Operation Test

3.5.1 Installation Plan

The manager shall ensure that the person/s in charge prepare an installation plan including, in principle, the following:

A.   Place of installation

B.   Timetable of installation

C.   Environment requirements recommended by the hardware supplier, such as temperature, humidity, vibration, etc.

D.   Installation conditions, such as power source, ground, etc.

E.   Title or name of the manager and person/s in charge

3.5.2 Installation of Hardware

A.   The person/s in charge shall install the hardware, ensure that it is appropriately installed, and keep a record in accordance with the installation plan.

B.   The manager shall evaluate the above and approve it thereafter.

3.5.3 Operation Test Plan

The manager shall ensure that the person/s in charge prepare an operation test (which shall thereafter mean every test for the evaluation of production and control performance under practical production conditions according to the specifications) plan, which shall include the following:

A.   Examination method for the function and capability of the system under operation

B.   Analysis and evaluation method for the test

3.5.4 Implementation of the Operation Test

A.   The person/s in charge shall conduct the operation test in accordance with the provisions of the operation test plan and keep a record of the test results.

B.   The manager shall evaluate the test results and thereafter approve it.

248   The Survive and Thrive Guide to Computer Validation

3.6   Others

All or part of the activities described in "development of the system" (see Part 3) can be entrusted to other firms on condition that the manufacturer concerned shall obtain and maintain the relevant documents of the activities from the contracting firm or otherwise ensure that these documents are properly retained by the contracting firm.

However, the contracted activities which fall within "System Performance Test" (see 3.4) or "Installation and Operation Test" (see 3.5) shall be directly supervised, evaluated, and accordingly approved by the responsible person designated by the manufacturer concerned.

Part 4: Operation Control

4.1   General

4.1.1   Responsibility of Operation

A.   The manufacturer shall designate a manager and person/s in charge for each of the operational steps prescribed in this part from "operation of hardware" (see 4.2) to "self-inspection" (see 4.6). The same person may also assume responsibility for several steps.

B.   The manager shall specify the duties of the person/s in charge.

4.1.2   Operation Procedures

The manufacturer shall prepare operations procedures including, in principle, the items shown below:

A.   Operation of the hardware

    a.   Standard operating procedures for the hardware

    b.   Education and training of personnel

B.   Inspection and maintenance

    a.   Periodic maintenance

        i.   Confirmation of appropriate program use

        ii.   Confirmation of system performance satisfying the function and capability descriptions in the specifications

        iii.   Necessary calibration of measuring instruments

GMP References, Electronic Records and Signatures 249

    b.   Daily inspection

        i.   Maintenance of the environment where the system operates

        ii.   Inspections before and after operation

        iii.   Inspection of entered data

    c.   Inspections to be carried out by specialists

C.   Countermeasures against accidents

    a.   Alarm setting of the system

    b.   System halt conditions

    c.   Personnel organization in case of accident

        i.   Organization chart

        ii.   Reporting system to the manager

    d.   Recovery procedures

    e.   Procedures for cause-finding studies

    f.   Procedures for the prevention of future accidents

    g.   Evaluation of the possible effects on products of the accidents or problems with the system

    h.   Procedures and check items for the resumption of operation after system shutdown

    i.   Procedures for necessary manual backup system

        i.   Scope of manually controlled devices

        ii.   Criteria for transfer to the manual system

        iii.   Evaluation of proper performance of manual system (including confirmation of relationship between both systems)

        iv.   Training for backup manual system

D.   Security control

    a   Restrictions for the hardware area

    b.   Designation of the person/s who are allowed to enter, modify or delete data, and the prevention of unauthorized data access

    c.   Control of passwords and identification codes

250   The Survive and Thrive Guide to Computer Validation

   i.   Registration, change and deletion procedures for passwords/identification codes

   ii.   Unauthorized opening of passwords/ identification codes

   iii. Security measures in case of changes in personnel authorized to use passwords/identification codes

d.   Programs and a set of data to be copied on a backup system, as well as provisions on the frequency of the renewal of the backup copies and storage condition

e.   Scope of activities of person/s in charge

E.   Title or name of the manager and person/s in charge of each step

4.1.3   System Alteration

A.   The manufacturer shall prepare a system alteration standard code which includes, in principle, the following:

a.   Procedures for alteration application and approval of alteration

b.   Examination after system alteration

c.   Amendment of operation procedures

d.   Notification of the amended parts to the persons concerned

e.   Title or name of the manager and person/s in charge

B.   The provisions ranging from "system engineering" (see 3.2) to "installation and operation test" (see 3.5) of Part 3, "development of the system" shall generally apply to the system alteration when associated with program change after its introduction.

4.2   Operation of Hardware

4.2.1   The manager shall ensure that person/s in charge operate the hardware in accordance with the standard operating procedures provided in the operations manual.

4.2.2   The manager shall train the person/s in charge based on the operating procedures.

4.3   Inspection and Maintenance

4.3.1   The person/s in charge shall implement inspection/maintenance in line with the provision of the operating procedures and keep a record of this.

4.3.2   The manager shall ensure that inspection/maintenance be properly undertaken based on the inspection/maintenance records.

GMP References, Electronic Records and Signatures   251

4.4 Accidents

4.4.1   The manager shall ensure that the person/s in charge take immediate actions when accidents occur in the system in accordance with the provisions of the operating procedures and let him/her conduct a cause-finding study as well as take necessary actions for the prevention of these accidents.

4.4.2   Resumption of operation may be allowed after the accidents on condition that the recovery is assured by the manager according to operating procedures.

4.4.3   The manager shall have the following records to be maintained by person/s in charge:

    A.   Contents and results of the accident

    B.   Records of cause-finding study and preventive measures

    C.   Confirmation by the manager

4.4.4   The manager shall ensure that a manual backup system be appropriately operated at the time of the accident in accordance with the operating procedure.

4.5 Security Control

4.5.1   The manager shall take necessary steps to prevent unauthorized persons from entering the computer area, in accordance with the operating procedures.

4.5.2   The manager should prevent unauthorized data access through designation of qualified person/s allowed to process data by entering, modifying, deleting, etc. according to the operating procedures.

4.5.3   The manager shall assume security control for passwords and identification codes in line with the operating procedures.

4.5.4   The person/s in charge shall provide a backup copy of the system and separately retain this in accordance with the provision of the operating procedures.

4.6 Self Inspection

4.6.1   The manufacturer shall ensure that the operation of the system is consonant with this guideline through periodic inspection by its manager.

4.6.2   The manager shall maintain a record of the self-inspection.

252   The Survive and Thrive Guide to Computer Validation

Part 5: Documentation (Including Plan, Procedures, and Others)

The manager shall retain the relevant documentation and records prepared according to this guideline in the following manner:

5.1 Methods

The following methods may be adopted:

A.   Paper printouts

B.   Magnetic tape or other methods. When this is applied, the following point shall be taken into account:

     a.   A backup copy shall be produced for documents and records.

     b.   Production and amendment of the documents and records shall be properly checked or recorded by the manager.

5.2 Storage Place

Documents and records relevant to the system development stage shall be maintained in each manufacturing premises concerned. All the documents may, however, be retained collectively on the major premises of the firm and copies concerned be distributed to each manufacturing location.

5.3 Storage Period

A.   Documents and records relevant to the system development stage shall be retained for three years from the date of retirement from operation of the system concerned (or, for one year after the expiry date in case of a drug required for labeling of the expiry date).

B.   Records relevant to system operation shall be retained for three years from the date of recording (or, for one year after the expiry date in case of a drug required for labeling of the expiry date).

Part 6: Date of Enforcement

This guideline shall be enforced on 1 Apr. 1993. The system already developed or under development on this date shall be exempted from this guideline.

U.S. FDA 21 CFR Part 11 Electronic Records; Electronic Signatures; Final Rule—Excerpts

Subpart B: Electronic Records

11.10   Controls for Closed Systems

Persons who use closed systems to create, modify, maintain, or transmit electronic records shall employ procedures and controls designed to ensure the authenticity, integrity, and, when appropriate, the confidentiality of electronic records, and to ensure that the signer cannot readily repudiate the signed record as not genuine. Such procedures and controls shall include the following:

a.   Validation of systems to ensure accuracy, reliability, consistent intended performance, and the ability to discern invalid or altered records.

b.   The ability to generate accurate and complete copies of records in both human readable and electronic form suitable for inspection, review, and copying by the agency.

c.   Protection of records to enable their accurate and ready retrieval throughout the records retention period.

d.   Limiting system access to authorized individuals.

e.   Use of secure, computer-generated, time-stamped audit trails to independently record the date and time of operator entries and actions that create, modify, or delete electronic records. Record changes shall not obscure previously recorded information. Such audit trail documentation shall be retained for a period at least as long as that required for the subject electronic records and shall be available for agency review and copying.

f.   Use of operational system checks to enforce permitted sequencing of steps and events, as appropriate.

g.   Use of authority checks to ensure that only authorized individuals can use the system, electronically sign a record, access the operation or computer system input or output device, alter a record, or perform the operation at hand.

h.   Use of device (e.g. terminal) checks to determine, as appropriate, the validity of the source of data input or operational instruction.

i.   Determination that persons who develop, maintain, or use electronic record/electronic signature systems have the education, raining, and experience to perform their assigned tasks.

254 The Survive and Thrive Guide to Computer Validation

j. The establishment of, and adherence to, written policies that hold individuals accountable and responsible for actions initiated under their electronic signatures, in order to deter record and signature falsification.

k. Use of appropriate controls over system documentation including:

1. Adequate controls over the distribution of, access to, and use of documentation for system operation and maintenance.

2. Revision and change control procedures to maintain an audit trail that documents time-sequenced development and modification of systems documentation.

11.30 Controls for Open Systems

Persons who use open system to create, modify, maintain, or transmit electronic records shall employ procedures and controls designed to ensure the authenticity, integrity, and, as appropriate, the confidentiality of electronic records from the point of their creation to the point of their receipt. Such procedures and controls shall include those identified in 21 CFR 11.10 as appropriate, and additional measures such as document encryption and use of appropriate digital signature standards to ensure, as necessary under the circumstances, record authenticity, integrity, and confidentiality.

11.50 Signature Manifestations

a. Signed electronic records shall contain information associated with the signing that clearly indicates all of the following:

1. The printed name of the signer;

2. The date and time when the signature was executed; and

3. The meaning (such as review, approval, responsibility, or authorship) associated with the signature.

b. The items identified in paragraphs a.1, a.2, and a.3 of this section shall be subject to the same controls as for electronic records and shall be included as part of any human-readable form of the electronic record (such as electronic display or printout).

11.70 Signature/Record Linking

Electronic signatures and handwritten signatures executed to electronic records shall be linked to their respective electronic records to ensure that the signatures cannot be excised, copied, or otherwise transferred to falsify an electronic records by ordinary means.

GMP References, Electronic Records and Signatures

Subpart C: Electronic Signatures

11.100 General Requirements

a. Each electronic signature shall be unique to one individual and shall not be reused by, or reassigned to, anyone else.

b. Before an organization establishes, assigns, certifies, or otherwise sanctions an individual's electronic signature, or any element of such electronic signature, the organization shall verify the identity of the individual.

c. Persons using electronic signatures shall, prior to or at the time of such use, certify to the agency that the electronic signatures in their system, used on or after August 20, 1997, are intended to be the legally binding equivalent of traditional handwritten signatures.

  1. The certification shall be submitted in paper form and signed with a traditional handwritten signature, to the Office of Regional Operations (HFC-100), 5600 Fishers Lane, Rockville, MD 20857.

  2. Persons using electronic signatures shall, upon agency request, provide additional certification or testimony that a specific electronic signature is the legally binding equivalent of the signer's handwritten signature.

11.200 Electronic Signature Components and Controls

a. Electronic signatures that are not based upon biometrics shall

  1. Employ at least two distinct identification components such as an identification code and a password.

    i. When an individual executes a series of signings during a single, continuous period of controlled system access, the first signing shall be executed using all electronic signature components; subsequent signings shall be executed using at least one electronic signature component that is only executable by, and designed to be used only by, the individual.

    ii. When an individual executes one or more signings not performed during a single, continuous period of controlled system access, each signing shall be executed using all of the electronic signature components.

  2. Be used only by their genuine owner; and

256   The Survive and Thrive Guide to Computer Validation

  3.   Be administered and executed to ensure that attempted use of an individual's electronic signature by anyone other than its genuine owner requires collaboration of two or more individuals.

b. Electronic signatures based upon biometrics shall be designed to ensure that they cannot be used by anyone other than their genuine owners.

11.300 Controls for Identification Codes/Passwords

Persons who use electronic signatures based upon use of identification codes in combination with passwords shall employ controls to ensure their security and integrity. Such controls shall include the following:

a. Maintaining the uniqueness of each combined identification code and password, so that no two individuals have the same combination of identification code and password.

b. Ensuring that identification code and password issuances are periodically checked, recalled, or revised (e.g., to cover such events as password aging).

c. Following loss management procedures to electronically deauthorize lost, stolen, missing, or otherwise compromised tokens, cards, and other devices that bear or generate identification code or password information, and to issue temporary or permanent replacements using suitable, rigorous controls.

d. Use of transaction safeguards to prevent unauthorized use of passwords and/or identification codes, and to detect and report in an immediate and urgent manner any attempts at their unauthorized use to system security unit, and, as appropriate, to organizational management.

e. Initial and periodic testing of devices, such as tokens and cards, that bear or generate identification code or password information to ensure that they function properly and have not been altered in an unauthorized manner.

14. OECD GLP and U.S. EPA GALP Excerpts

Introduction—Document Contacts

In this chapter, there are excerpts from two directives for good practices with laboratory systems. Experience has shown that these documents are very useful for adapting to the practical work of computer validation. Original copies of these documents may be acquired through their regulatory sources.

Organization for Economic Cooperation and Development (OECD)

> Head of Publications Service
> OECD
> 2 rue Andre-Pascal
> 75775 Paris Cedex 16, FRANCE

U.S. Environmental Protection Agency (EPA)

> Scientific Systems Staff
> Office of Information resources Management
> U.S. Environmental Protection Agency
> Research Triangle Park, North Carolina 27711

258　The Survive and Thrive Guide to Computer Validation

GLP Consensus Document: The Application of the Principles of GLP to Computerized Systems—OECD, Paris, 1995

Source: OECD Series on Principles of Good Laboratory Practice and Compliance Monitoring, Number 10, Environment Monograph No. 116. OECD Environment Directorate, Paris, 1995.

Throughout recent years there has been an increase in the use of computerized systems by test facilities undertaking health and environmental safety testing. These computerized systems may be involved with the direct or indirect capture of data, processing, reporting and storage of data, and increasingly as an integral part of automated equipment. Where these computerized systems are associated with the conduct of studies intended for regulatory purposes, it is essential that they are developed, validated, operated and maintained in accordance with the OECD Principles of Good Laboratory Practice (GLP).

Scope

All computerized systems used for the generation, measurement or assessment of data intended for regulatory submission should be developed, validated, operated and maintained in ways which are compliant with the GLP Principles.

During the planning, conduct and reporting of studies, there may be several computerized systems in use for a variety of purposes. Such purposes might include the direct or indirect capture of data from automated instruments, operation/control of automated equipment and the processing, reporting and storage of data. For these different activities, computerized systems can vary from a programmable analytical instrument or a personal computer to a laboratory information management system (LIMS) with multiple functions. Whatever the scale of computer involvement, the GLP Principles should be applied.

Approach

Computerized systems associated with the conduct of studies destined for regulatory submission should be of appropriate design, adequate capacity and suitable for their intended purposes. There should be appropriate procedures to control and maintain these systems, and the systems should be developed, validated and operated in a way which is in compliance with the GLP Principles. The demonstration that a computerized system is suitable for its intended purpose is of fundamental importance and is referred to as computer validation.

The validation process provides a high degree of assurance that a computerized system meets its pre-determined specifications. Validation should be undertaken by means of a formal validation plan and performed prior to operational use.

The Application of the GLP Principles to Computerized Systems

The following considerations will assist in the application of the GLP Principles to computerized systems outlined above:

1. Responsibilities

a. *Management* of a test facility has the overall responsibility for compliance with the GLP Principles. This responsibility includes the appointment and effective organization of an adequate number of appropriately qualified and experienced staff, as well as the obligation to ensure that the facilities, equipment and data handling procedures are of an adequate standard.

Management is responsible for ensuring that computerized systems are suitable for their intended purposes. It should establish computing policies and procedures to ensure that systems are developed, validated, operated and maintained in accordance with the GLP Principles. Management should also ensure that these policies and procedures are understood and followed, and ensure that effective monitoring of such requirements occurs.

Management should also designate personnel with specific responsibility for the development, validation, operation and maintenance of computerized systems. Such personnel should be suitably qualified, with relevant experience and appropriate training to perform their duties in accordance with the GLP Principles.

b. *Study Directors* are responsible under the GLP Principles for the overall conduct of their studies. Since many such studies will utilize computerized systems, it is essential that Study Directors are fully aware of the involvement of any computerized systems used in studies under their direction.

The Study Director's responsibility for data recorded electronically is the same as that for data recorded on paper and thus only systems that have been validated should be used in GLP studies.

c. *Personnel.* All personnel using computerized systems have a responsibility for operating these systems in compliance with the GLP Principles. Personnel who develop, validate, operate and maintain computerized systems are responsible

260   The Survive and Thrive Guide to Computer Validation

for performing such activities in accordance with the GLP Principles and recognized technical standards.

d. *Quality Assurance* (QA) responsibilities for computerized systems must be defined by management and described in written policies and procedures. The quality assurance program should include procedures and practices that will assure that established standards are met for all phases of the validation, operation and maintenance of computerized systems. It should also include procedures and practices for the introduction of purchased systems and for the process of in-house development of computerized systems.

Quality Assurance personnel are required to monitor the GLP compliance of computerized systems and should be given training in any specialist techniques necessary. They should be sufficiently familiar with such systems so as to permit objective comment; in some cases the appointment of specialist auditors may be necessary.

QA personnel should have, for review, direct read-only access to the data stored within a computerized system.

2. Training

The GLP Principles require that a test facility has appropriately qualified and experienced personnel and that there are documented training programs, including both on-the-job training and, where appropriate, attendance an external training courses. Records of all such training should be maintained.

The above provisions should also apply for all personnel involved with computerized systems.

3. Facilities and Equipment

Adequate facilities and equipment should be available for the proper conduct of studies in compliance with GLP. For computerized systems there will be a number of specified considerations:

a. Facilities

Due consideration should be given to the physical location of computer hardware, peripheral components, communications equipment and electronic storage media. Extremes of temperature and humidity, dust, electromagnetic interference and proximity to high voltage cables should be avoided unless the equipment is specifically designed to operate under such conditions.

Consideration must also be given to the electrical supply for computer equipment and, where appropriate, backup or uninterruptable supplies for computerized systems, whose sudden failure would affect the results of a study.

Adequate facilities should be provided for the secure retention of electronic storage media.

b. Equipment

i. Hardware and Software

A computerized system is defined as a group of hardware components and associated software designed and assembled to perform a specific function or group of functions.

Hardware is the physical components of the computerized system; it will include the computer unit itself and its peripheral components.

Software is the program or programs that control the operation of the computerized system.

All GLP Principles which apply to equipment therefore apply to both hardware and software.

ii. Communications

Communications related to computerized systems broadly fall into two categories: between computers or between computers and peripheral components.

All communication links are potential sources of error and may result in the loss or corruption of data. Appropriate controls for security and system integrity must be adequately addressed during the development, validation, operation and maintenance of any computerized system.

4. Maintenance and Disaster Recovery

All computerized systems should be installed and maintained in a manner to ensure the continuity of accurate performance.

a. Maintenance

There should be documented procedures covering both routine preventative maintenance and fault repair. These procedures should clearly detail the roles and

262 The Survive and Thrive Guide to Computer Validation

responsibilities of personnel involved. Where such maintenance activities have necessitated changes to hardware and/or software, it may be necessary to validate the system again. During the daily operation of the system, records should be maintained of any problems or inconsistencies detected and any remedial action taken.

b. Disaster Recovery

Procedures should be in place describing the measures to be taken in the event of partial or total failure of a computerized system. Measures may range from planned hardware redundancy to transition back to a paper-based system. All contingency plans need to be well documented, validated, and should ensure continued data integrity and should not compromise the study in any way. Personnel involved in the conduct of studies according to the GLP Principles should be aware of such contingency plans.

Procedures for the recovery of a computerized system will depend on the criticality of the system, but it is essential that backup copies of all software are maintained. If recovery procedures entail changes to hardware or software, it may be necessary to validate the system again.

5. Data

The GLP Principles define raw data as being all original laboratory records and documentation, including data directly entered into a computer through an instrument interface, which are the results of original observations and activities in a study and which are necessary for the reconstruction and evaluation of the report of that study.

Computerized systems operating in compliance with GLP Principles may be associated with raw data in a variety of forms, for example, electronic storage media, computer or instrument printouts and microfilm/fiche copies. It is necessary that raw data are defined for each computerized system.

Where computerized systems are used to capture, process, report or store raw date electronically, system design should always provide for the retention of full audit trails to show all changes to the data without obscuring the original data. It should be possible to associate all changes to data with the persons making those changes by use of timed and dated (electronic) signatures. Reasons for change should be given.

OECD GLP and U.S. EPA GALP Excerpts   263

When raw data are held electronically, it is necessary to provide for long-term retention requirements for the type of data held and the expected life of computerized systems. Hardware and software system changes must provide for continued access to and retention of the raw data without integrity risks.

Supporting information such as maintenance logs and calibration records that are necessary to verify the validity of raw data or to permit reconstruction of a process or a study should be retained in the archives.

Procedures for the operation of a computerized system should also describe the alternative data capture procedures to be followed in the event of system failure. In such circumstances, any manually recorded raw data subsequently entered into the computer should be clearly identified as such, and should be retained as the original record. Manual backup procedures should serve to minimize the risk of any data loss and ensure that these alternative records are retained.

Where system obsolescence forces a need to transfer electronic raw data from one system to another then the process must be well documented and its integrity verified. Where such migration is not practicable, then the raw data must be transferred to another medium and this verified as an exact copy prior to any destruction of the original electronic records.

6. Security

Documented security procedures should be in place for the protection of hardware, software and data from corruption or unauthorized modification, or loss. In this context security includes the prevention of unauthorized access or changes to the computerized system, as well as to the data held within the system. The potential for corruption of data by viruses or other agents should also be addressed. Security measures should also be taken to ensure data integrity in the event of both short-term and long-term system failure.

a. Physical Security

Physical security measures should be in place to restrict access to computer hardware, communications equipment, peripheral components and electronic storage media to authorized personnel only. For equipment not held within specific "computer rooms" (e.g., personal computers and terminals), standard test facility access controls are necessary as a minimum. However, where such equipment is located remotely (e.g., portable components and modem links), additional measures need to be taken.

264   The Survive and Thrive Guide to Computer Validation

b. Logical Security

For each computerized system or application, logical security measures must be in place to prevent unauthorized access to the computerized system, applications and data. It is essential to ensure that only approved versions and validated software are in use. Logical security may include the need to enter a unique user identity with an associated password. Any introduction of data or software from external sources should be controlled. These controls may be provided by the computer operating system software, by specific security routines, routines embedded into the applications, or combinations of the above.

c. Data Integrity

Since maintaining data integrity is a primary objective of the GLP Principles, it is important that everyone associated with a computerized system is aware of the necessity for the above security considerations. Management should ensure that personnel are aware of the importance of data security, the procedures and system features that are available to provide appropriate security and the consequences of security breaches. Such system features could include routine surveillance of system access, the implementation of file verification routines and exception and/or trend reporting.

d. Backup

It is standard practice with computerized systems to make backup copies of all software and data to allow for recovery of the system following any failure which compromises the integrity of the system, e.g., disk corruption. The implication, therefore, is that the backup copy may become raw data and must be treated as such.

7. Validation of Computerized Systems

Computerized systems must be suitable for their intended purpose. The following aspects should be addressed:

a. Acceptance

Computerized systems should be designed to satisfy GLP Principles and introduced in a pre-planned manner. There should be adequate documentation that each system was developed in a controlled manner and preferably according to quality and technical standards (e.g., ISO/9001). Furthermore, there should be evidence that the system was adequately tested for conformance with the acceptance criteria by the test facility prior to being put into routine use. Formal acceptance testing requires the conduct of tests following a pre-defined plan and retention of documented evidence of all testing procedures, test data, test results, a formal summary of testing and a record of formal acceptance.

For vendor-supplied systems, it is likely that much of the documentation created during the development is retained at the vendor's site. In this case, evidence of formal assessment and/or vendor audits should be available at the test facility.

b. Retrospective Evaluation

There will be systems where the need for compliance with GLP Principles was not foreseen or not specified. Where this occurs, there should be documented justification for use of the systems; this should involve a retrospective evaluation to assess suitability.

Retrospective evaluation begins by gathering all historical records related to the computerized system. These records are then reviewed and a written summary is produced. This retrospective evaluation summary should specify what validation evidence is available and what needs to be done in the future to ensure validation of the computerized system.

c. Change Control

Change control is the formal approval and documentation of any change to the computerized system during the operational life of the system. Change control is needed when a change may affect the computerized system's validation status. Change control procedures must be effective once the computerized system is operational.

The procedure should describe the method of evaluation to determine the extent of retesting necessary to maintain the validated state of the system. The change control procedure should identify the persons responsible for determining the necessity for change control and its approval.

Irrespective of the origin of the change (supplier or in-house developed system), appropriate information needs to be provided as part of the change control process. Change control procedures should ensure data integrity.

d. Support Mechanism

In order to ensure that a computerized system remains suitable for its intended purpose, support mechanisms should be in place to ensure the system is functioning and being used correctly. This may involve system management, training,

266   The Survive and Thrive Guide to Computer Validation

maintenance, technical support, auditing and/or performance assessment. Performance assessment is the formal review of a system at periodic intervals to ensure that it continues to meet stated performance criteria, e.g., reliability, responsiveness, capacity.

8. Documentation

The items listed below are a guide to the minimum documentation for the development, validation, operation and maintenance of computerized systems.

a. Policies

There should be written management policies covering, *inter alia*, the acquisition, requirements, design, validation, testing, installation, operation, maintenance, staffing, control, auditing, monitoring and retirement of computerized systems.

b. Application Description

For each application there should be documentation fully describing:

- The name of the application software or identification code and a detailed and clear description of the purpose of the application.

- The hardware (with model numbers) on which the application software operates.

- The operating system and other system software (e.g., tools) used in conjunction with the application.

- The application programming language(s) and/or database tools used.

- The major functions performed by the application.

- An overview of the type and flow of data/database design associated with the application.

- File structures, error and alarm message, and algorithms associated with the application.

- The application software components with version numbers.

- Configuration and communication links among application modules and to equipment and other systems.

c. Source Code

Some OECD Member countries require that the source code for application software should be available at, or retrievable to, the test facility.

OECD GLP and U.S. EPA GALP Excerpts   267

d. Standard Operating Procedures (SOPs)

Much of the documentation covering the use of computerized systems will be in the form of SOPs. These should cover but not be limited to the following:

- Procedures for the operation of computerized systems (hardware/software), and the responsibilities of personnel involved.

- Procedures for security measures used to detect and prevent unauthorized access and program changes.

- Procedures and authorization for program changes and the recording of changes.

- Procedures and authorization for changes to equipment (hardware/software) including testing before use if appropriate.

- Procedures for the periodic testing for correct functioning of the complete system or its component parts and the recording of these tests.

- Procedures for the maintenance of computerized systems and any associated equipment.

- Procedures for software development and acceptance testing, and the recording of all acceptance testing.

- Backup procedures for all stored data and contingency plans in the event of a breakdown.

- Procedures for the archiving and retrieval of all documents, software and computer data.

- Procedures for the monitoring and auditing of computerized systems.

9. Archives

The GLP Principles for archiving data must be applied consistently to all data types. It is therefore important that electronic data are stored with the same levels of access control, indexing and expedient retrieval as other types of data.

Where electronic data from more than one study are stored on a single storage medium (e.g., disk or tape), a detailed index will be required.

It may be necessary to provide facilities with specific environmental controls appropriate to ensure the integrity of the stored electronic data. If this necessitates additional archive facilities then management should ensure that the personnel responsible for managing the archives are identified and that access is limited to authorized personnel. It will also be necessary to implement procedures to ensure that the long-term integrity of data stored electronically is not compromised. Where problems with long-term access to data are envisaged or when computerized

268 The Survive and Thrive Guide to Computer Validation

systems have to be retired, procedures for ensuring that continued readability of the data should be established. This may, for example, include producing hard copy printouts or transferring the data to another system.

No electronically stored data should be destroyed without management authorization and relevant documentation. Other data held in support of computerized systems, such as source code and development, validation, operation, maintenance and monitoring records, should be held for at least as long as study records associated with these systems.

Definition of Terms

Acceptance Criteria: The documented criteria that should be met to successfully complete a test phase or to meet delivery requirements

Acceptance Testing: Formal testing of a computerized system in its anticipated operating environment to determine whether all acceptance criteria of the test facility have been met and whether the system is acceptable for operational use.

Backup: Provisions made for the recovery of data files or software, for the restart of processing, or for the use of alternative computer equipment after a system failure or disaster.

Change Control: Ongoing evaluation and documentation of system operations and changes to determine whether a validation process is necessary following any changes to the computerized system.

Computerized System: A group of hardware components and associated software designed and assembled to perform a specific function or group of functions.

Electronic Signature: The entry in the form of magnetic impulses or computer data compilation of any symbol or series of symbols, executed, adapted or authorized by a person to be equivalent to the person's handwritten signature.

Hardware: The physical components of a computerized system, including the computer unit itself and its peripheral components.

Peripheral Components: Any interfaced instrumentation, or auxiliary or remote components such as printers, modems and terminals, etc.

Recognized Technical Standards: Standards as promulgated by national or international standard setting bodies (ISO, IEEE, ANSI, etc.)

OECD GLP and U.S. EPA GALP Excerpts   269

Security: The protection of computer hardware and software from accidental or malicious access, use, modification, destruction or disclosure. Security also pertains to personnel, data, communications and the physical and logical protection of computer installations.

Software (Application): A program acquired for or developed, adapted or tailored to the test facility requirements for the purpose of controlling processes, data collection, data manipulation, data reporting and/or archiving.

Software (Operating System): A program or collection of programs, routines and subroutines that controls the operation of a computer. An operating system may provide services such as resource allocation, scheduling, input/output control, and data management.

Source Code: An original computer program expressed in human-readable form (programming language) which must be translated into machine-readable form before it can be executed by the computer.

Validation of a Computerized System: The demonstration that a computerized system is suitable for its intended purpose.

270   **The Survive and Thrive Guide to Computer Validation**

EPA 2185—Good Automated Laboratory Practices (GALP)

Source: U.S. Environmental Protection Agency (EPA) GALP: Principles and Guidance to Regulations for Ensuring Data Integrity in Automated Laboratory Operations with Implementation Guidance—1995 Edition. Only the Scope and Section 8 from Chapter 1 of the GALP document are included here. Chapter 2 is very useful and contains 128 pages of practical advice on how to implement the GALPs, but is not included.

Scope

Applicable Systems

The GALPs use the acronym LIMS, laboratory information management system, to describe the automated laboratory systems that collect and manage data discussed in this Directive. There is a limitless range of possible configurations of automated data collection and processing equipment, communication components, types of operating system software, database management systems, and application software that can constitute a LIMS. The GALPs are directed to *most* configurations that are involved with entering, recording, manipulating, modifying, and retrieving data.

Not all laboratory systems are LIMS. Automated laboratory systems that record data but do not allow changes to the data are not LIMS. For example, an instrument that measures weights and produces or maintains a readout of the weight is not a LIMS, if the true reading cannot be altered by a person prior to recording.

The ability to effect changes to original observations or measurements is the factor in determining whether the automated laboratory system is a LIMS. If data entering automated laboratory systems can be manipulated or changed in any way by the action of a person prior to being recorded, then that automated laboratory system is a LIMS.

8. Good Automated Laboratory Practices

8.1   Laboratory Management

When LIMS Raw Data (see 8.4.1) are collected, analyzed, processed, or maintained, laboratory management shall:

8.1.1   ensure that personnel clearly understand the function(s) they are to perform on the LIMS.

OECD GLP and U.S. EPA GALP Excerpts 271

8.1.2 ensure that a Quality Assurance Unit (QAU) monitors LIMS activities as described in 8.3.

8.1.3 ensure that personnel, resources, and facilities are adequate and available as scheduled.

8.1.4 receive reports of QAU of inspections of the LIMS (see 8.3.3) and audits of LIMS Raw Data (see 8.3.5) and ensure that corrective actions are promptly taken in response to any deficiencies.

8.1.5 approve the standard operating procedures (SOPs), setting forth the methods that assure LIMS Raw Data integrity, ensure that any deviations from SOPs and applicable GALP provisions are appropriately documented and that corrective actions are taken and documented, and approve subsequent changes to SOPs (see 8.11).

8.1.6 assure that each applicable GALP provision is followed. With the exception of 8.1, 8.2, and 8.3, laboratory management may delegate GALP implementation and compliance to one or more responsible persons.

8.2 Personnel

When LIMS Raw Data are collected, analyzed, processed, or maintained, laboratory management shall ensure that all LIMS support staff and users:

8.2.1 have adequate education, training, and experience to perform assigned LIMS functions.

8.2.2 have a current summary of their training, experience, and job description, including their knowledge relevant to LIMS design and operation, maintained at the facility.

8.2.3 are of sufficient number for timely and proper operation of the LIMS.

8.3 Quality Assurance Unit

When LIMS Raw Data are collected, analyzed, processed, or maintained, laboratory management shall designate a Quality Assurance Unit (QAU) to monitor LIMS functions and procedures. The QAU shall:

8.3.1 be entirely separate from and independent of LIMS personnel, and shall report directly to laboratory management.

8.3.2 have immediate access to the LIMS data, SOPs, and other records pertaining to the operation and maintenance of the LIMS.

8.3.3 inspect the LIMS at intervals adequate to ensure the integrity of the LIMS Raw Data (see 8.3.5); prepare inspection reports that include a description

272 The Survive and Thrive Guide to Computer Validation

of the LIMS operation inspected, the dates of the inspection, the person performing the inspection, findings and problems observed, action recommended and taken to resolve existing problems, and any scheduled dates for reinspection; and report to laboratory management any problems that may affect data integrity.

8.3.4 determine that no deviations from approved SOPs were made without proper authorization (see 8.1.5) and sufficient documentation.

8.3.5 periodically audit the LIMS Raw Data to ensure their integrity.

8.3.6 ensure that the responsibilities and procedures applicable to the QAU, the records maintained by the QAU, and the method of indexing such records are documented and are maintained.

8.4 LIMS Raw Data

Laboratory management shall ensure that:

8.4.1 LIMS Raw Data (LRD) and LRD storage media on which they reside (see 9. Definitions LIMS Raw Data and LIMS Raw Data Storage media) are identified and documented. This documentation shall be included in the laboratory's SOPs.

8.4.2 the individual(s) responsible for entering and recording LIMS Raw Data are uniquely identified when the data are recorded, and the time(s) and date(s) are documented.

8.4.3 the instrument transmitting LIMS Raw Data is uniquely identified when the data are recorded, and the time and date are documented.

8.4.4 procedures and practices to verify the accuracy of LIMS Raw Data are documented and included in the laboratory's SOPs, and managed as described in 8.11.

8.4.5 procedures and practices for making changes to LIMS Raw Data are documented and provide evidence of change, preserve the original recorded documentation (see 8.4.2 and 8.4.3), are dated, indicate the reason for the change, identify the person who made the change and, if different, the person who authorized the change. These procedures shall be included in the laboratory's SOPs, and managed as described in 8.11.

8.5 Software

When software is used to collect, analyze, process, or maintain LIMS Raw Data, laboratory management shall ensure that:

8.5.1 SOPs are established, approved, and managed as described in 8.11 for:

OECD GLP and U.S. EPA GALP Excerpts   273

8.5.1.1 development methodologies that are based on the size and nature of software being developed. EPA and its agents shall comply with *EPA Information Resources Management Policy Manual Chapter 17.*

8.5.1.2 testing and quality assurance methods to ensure that all LIMS software accurately performs its intended functions, including: acceptance criteria, test to be used, personnel responsible for conducting the tests, documentation of test results, and test review and approval.

8.5.1.3 change control methods that include instructions for requesting, testing, approving, documenting, and implementing changes. When indicated, change control methods shall also include reporting and evaluating problems, as well as implementing corrective actions.

8.5.1.4 version control methods that document the LIMS software version currently used.

8.5.1.5 maintaining a historical file of software, software operating procedures (manuals), software changes, and software version numbers.

8.5.2 documentation is established and maintained to demonstrate the validity of software used in the LIMS:

8.5.2.1 for existing and commercially available LIMS, minimum documentation shall include, but not be limited to: a description of the software and functional requirements; listing of all algorithms and formulas; and, as they occur, testing and quality assurance, installation and operation, maintenance/enhancement, and retirement.

8.5.2.2 for new LIMS development or modification of existing LIMS, documentation shall cover all phases of the generic software life cycle. EPA laboratories and those of its agents (contractors and grantees) shall comply with the documentation requirements specified in *EPA Information Resources Management Policy Manual Chapter 17.*

8.5.3 all documentation specified in 8.5.2 is readily available in the facility where the software is used, and the SOPs specified in 8.5.1 are readily available in the laboratory areas where procedures are performed.

8.5.4 a historical file of software and the documentation specified in 8.5.2 are retained according to procedures outlined in 8.9.

8.6 Security

Laboratory management shall ensure that security practices to assure the integrity of LIMS data are adequate. EPA laboratories and those of its agents (contractors and grantees) shall comply with EPA's Information Security Policy.

274   The Survive and Thrive Guide to Computer Validation

8.7   Hardware

When LIMS Raw Data are collected, analyzed, processed, or maintained, laboratory management shall ensure that LIMS hardware and communications components are

8.7.1   of adequate design and capacity, and a description is documented and maintained.

8.7.2   installed and operated in accordance with manufacturer's recommendations and, at installation, under-go acceptance testing that conforms to acceptance criteria. SOPs shall be established and maintained to define the acceptance criteria, testing, documentation, and approval required for changes to LIMS hardware and communications components.

8.7.3   adequately tested, inspected, and maintained. SOPs for and documentation of these routine operations shall be maintained. Documentation of non-routine maintenance shall also include a description of the problem, the corrective action, acceptance testing criteria, and the acceptance testing performed to ensure that the LIMS hardware and communications components have been adequately repaired.

8.8   Comprehensive Testing

When LIMS Raw Data are collected, analyzed, processed, or maintained, laboratory management shall ensure that comprehensive testing of LIMS performance is conducted at least every 24 months or more frequently as a result of software (see 8.5.2) or hardware (see 8.7.2) changes or modifications. These tests shall be documented and the documentation shall be retained and available for inspection or audit.

8.9   Records Retention

Laboratory management shall ensure that retention of LIMS Raw Data, documentation, and records pertaining to the LIMS comply with EPA contract, statute, or regulation; and SOPs for retention are documented, maintained, and managed as described in 8.11.

8.10   Facilities

When LIMS Raw Data are collected, analyzed, processed, or maintained, laboratory management shall ensure that:

8.10.1   the environmental conditions of the facility housing the LIMS are regulated to protect against LIMS Raw Data loss.

OECD GLP and U.S. EPA GALP Excerpts 275

    8.10.2 environmentally adequate storage capability for retention of LIMS Raw Data, LIMS Raw Data storage media, documentation, and records pertaining to the LIMS are provided.

8.11 Standard Operating Procedures

Laboratory management shall ensure that:

    8.11.1 SOPs include, but are not limited to, those specified in 8.4.1, 8.4.4, 8.4.5, 8.5.1.1 through 8.5.1.5, 8.7.2, 8.7.3, and 8.9. Each current SOP shall be readily available where the procedure is performed.

    8.11.2 SOPs are periodically reviewed at a frequency adequate to ensure that they accurately describe the current procedures.

    8.11.3 SOPs are authorized and changed in accordance with 8.1.5.

    8.11.4 A historical file of SOPs is maintained.

9.   Definitions—Excerpts

LIMS Raw Data (LRD)—Original observations recorded by the LIMS that are needed to verify, calculate, or derive data that are or may be reported.

LIMS Raw Data (LRD) storage media—The media to which LIMS Raw Data are first recorded.

Original observations—The first occurrence of human-readable information.

Software life cycle—The period of time beginning when a software product is conceived and ending when the product no longer performs the function for which it was designed. The software life cycle is typically broken into phases, such as initiation, requirements analysis, design, programming, testing and quality assurance, installation and operation, maintenance, and retirement.

15. ICH and FDA Guidelines for GCP Systems—Excerpts

Introduction—Document Sources

This chapter references two document of GCP importance. The first has excerpts from the ICH GCP that are relevant to the use of computerized systems in clinical studies. The second document has all of the text of the FDA draft guideline for computer systems used in clinical trials.

While the ICH document has only certain portions of it relevant to electronic systems, it is an official regulation for all trials conducted in the Member States of the European Union as of January 17, 1997. The FDA Guideline, in contrast, is a draft document and published for comment and review by industry at the time this book goes to press. It is included herein to give the reader a view of the current thinking of FDA about the quality assurance of GCP systems.

A copy of the original full text of both documents may be acquired over the Internet from the U.S. FDA home page.

U.S. Food and Drug Administration (FDA)

All US and ICH regulatory documents are available through the FDA's Internet home page at http://www.fda.gov in the Guidance Index.

Other documents useful to computer validation activities are available from the FDA home page and can be found in the *Guidance for Industry Index*. One such document is the following:

278   The Survive and Thrive Guide to Computer Validation

General Principles of Software Validation—Draft Guidance Version 1.1

Released for comment on: June 9, 1997

This document outlines general validation principles that FDA considers applicable to the validation of medical device software or the validation of software used to design, develop, or manufacture medical devices.

ICH and FDA Guidelines for GCP Systems—Excerpts 279

ICH GCP—Computer Relevant Excerpts

Source: Excerpts from the International Conference on Harmonization (ICH) GCP adopted by the EMEA and published in the Federal Register by the U.S. FDA.

ICH Topic E6—Guideline for Good Clinical Practice—EMEA— for Trials Starting After January 17, 1997

Introduction

Good Clinical Practice (GCP) is an international ethical and scientific quality standard for designing, conducting, recording and reporting trials that involve the participation of human subjects. Compliance with this standard provides public assurance that the rights, safety and well-being of trial subjects are protected, consistent with the principles that have their origin in the Declaration of Helsinki, and that the clinical trial data are credible.

The objective of this ICH GCP Guideline is to provide a unified standard for the European Union (EU), Japan and the United States to facilitate the mutual acceptance of clinical data by the regulatory authorities in these jurisdictions.

The guideline was developed with consideration of the current good clinical practices of the European Union, Japan, and the United States, as well as those of Australia, Canada, the Nordic countries and the World Health Organization (WHO).

1.   *Glossary (Subset of Terms Relevant to Electronic Systems)*

1.6   **Audit**—A systematic and independent examination of trial-related activities and documents to determine whether the evaluated trial-related activities were conducted, and the data were recorded, analyzed and accurately reported according to the protocol, sponsor's standard operating procedures (SOPs), Good Clinical Practice (GCP), and the applicable regulatory requirement(s).

1.9   **Audit Trail**—Documentation that allows reconstruction of the course of events.

1.11   **Case Report Form (CRF)**—A printed, optical, or electronic document designed to record all of the protocol-required information to be reported to the sponsor on each trial subject.

1.22   **Documentation**—All records, in any form (including, but not limited to, written, electronic, magnetic, and optical records, and scans, x-rays, and

280 The Survive and Thrive Guide to Computer Validation

electrocardiograms) that describe or record the methods, conduct, and/or results of a trial, the factors affecting a trial, and the actions taken.

1.24 **Good Clinical Practice (GCP)**—A standard for the design, conduct, performance, monitoring, auditing, recording, analyses, and reporting of clinical trials that provides assurance that the data and reported results are credible and accurate, and that the rights, integrity, and confidentiality of trial subjects are protected.

1.38 **Monitoring**—The act of overseeing the progress of a clinical trial, and of ensuring that it is conducted, recorded, and reported in accordance with the protocol, Standard Operating Procedures (SOPs), Good Clinical Practice (GCP), and the applicable regulatory requirement(s).

1.43 **Original Medical Record**—See Source Document.

1.51 **Source Data**—All information in original records and certified copies of original records of clinical findings, observations, or other activities in a clinical trial necessary for the reconstruction and evaluation of the trial. Source data are contained in source documents (original records or certified copies).

1.52 **Source Documents**—Original documents, data, and records (e.g., hospital records, clinical and office charts, laboratory notes, memoranda, subjects' diaries or evaluation checklists, pharmacy dispensing records, recorded data from automated instruments, copies or transcriptions certified after verification as being accurate copies, microfiches, photographic negatives, microfilm or magnetic media, x-rays, subject files, and records kept at the pharmacy, at the laboratories and at medico-technical departments involved in the clinical trial).

2. *The Principles of ICH GCP*

2.8 Each individual involved in conducting a trial should be qualified by education, training, and experience to perform his or her respective task(s).

2.10 All clinical trial information should be recorded, handled, and stored in a way that allows its accurate reporting, interpretation and verification.

2.13 Systems with procedures that assure the quality of every aspect of the trial should be implemented.

ICH and FDA Guidelines for GCP Systems—Excerpts   281

4. *Investigator*

4.9   Records and Reports

4.9.1   The investigator should ensure the accuracy, completeness, legibility, and timeliness of the data reported to the sponsor in the CRFs and in all reports.

4.9.2   Data reported on the CRF that are derived from source documents should be consistent with the source documents or the discrepancies should be explained.

4.9.3   Any change or correction to a CRF should be dated, initialed, and explained (if necessary) and should not obscure the original entry (i.e. an audit trail should be maintained); this applies to both written and electronic changes or corrections (see 5.18.4(n)). Sponsors should provide guidance to investigators and/or the investigators' designated representatives on making such corrections. Sponsors should have written procedures to assure that changes or corrections in CRFs made by sponsor's designated representatives are documented, are necessary, and are endorsed by the investigator. The investigator should retain records of the changes and corrections.

4.9.5   Essential documents should be retained until at least 2 years after the last approval of a marketing authorization application in an ICH region and until there are no pending or contemplated marketing applications in an ICH region or at least 2 years have elapsed since the formal discontinuation of clinical development of the investigational product.

5. *Sponsor*

5.1   Quality Assurance and Quality Control

5.1.1   The sponsor is responsible for implementing and maintaining quality assurance and quality control systems with written SOPs to ensure that trials are conducted and data are generated, documented (recorded), and reported in compliance with the protocol, GCP, and the applicable regulatory requirement(s).

5.1.3   Quality control should be applied to each stage of data handling to ensure that all data are reliable and have been processed correctly.

5.2   Contract Research Organizations (CRO)

5.2.1   A sponsor may transfer any or all of the sponsor's trial-related duties and functions to a CRO, but the ultimate responsibility for the quality and

282   The Survive and Thrive Guide to Computer Validation

integrity of the trial data always resides with the sponsor. The CRO should implement quality assurance and quality control.

5.2.2   Any trial-related duty and function that is transferred to and assumed by a CRO should be specified in writing.

5.5   Trial Management, Data Handling, and Recordkeeping

5.5.1   The sponsor should utilize appropriately qualified individuals to supervise the overall conduct of the trial, to handle the data, to verify the data, conduct the statistical analyses, and to prepare the trial reports.

5.5.3   When using electronic trial data handling and/or remote electronic trial data systems, the sponsor should:

    a.   Ensure and document that the electronic data processing system(s) conforms to the sponsor's established requirements for completeness, accuracy, reliability, and consistent intended performance (i.e., validation).

    b.   Maintain SOPs for using these systems.

    c.   Ensure that the systems are designed to permit data changes in such a way that the data changes are documented and that there is no deletion of entered data (i.e., maintain an audit trail, data trail, edit trail).

    d.   Maintain a security system that prevents unauthorized access to the data.

    e.   Maintain a list of the individuals who are authorized to make data changes (see 4.1.5 and 4.9.3).

    f.   Maintain adequate backup of the data.

    g.   Safeguard the blinding, if any (e.g. maintain the blinding during data entry and processing).

5.5.4   If data are transformed during processing, it should always be possible to compare the original data and observations with the processed data.

5.6   Investigator Selection

5.6.1   The sponsor is responsible for selecting the investigator(s)/institution(s). Each investigator should be qualified by training and experience and should have adequate resources (see 4.1,4.2) to properly conduct the trial for which the investigator is selected.

5.6.3   The sponsor should obtain the investigator's/institution's agreements:

ICH and FDA Guidelines for GCP Systems—Excerpts   283

a.   to conduct the trial in compliance with GCP, with the applicable regulatory requirement(s) (see 4.1.3), and with the protocol agreed to by the sponsor and given approval/favorable opinion by the IRB/IEC (see 4.5.1);

b.   to comply with procedures for data recording/reporting;

c.   to permit monitoring, auditing and inspection (see 4.1.4) and

d.   to retain the trial related essential documents until the sponsor informs the investigator/institution these documents are no longer needed (see 4.9.4 and 5.5.12).

The sponsor and the investigator/institution should sign the protocol, or an alternative document, to confirm this agreement.

5.18   Monitoring

5.18.4 Monitor's Responsibilities

The monitor(s) in accordance with the sponsor's requirements should ensure that the trial is conducted and documented properly by carrying out the following activities when relevant and necessary to the trial and the trial site:

a.   Acting as the main line of communication between the sponsor and the investigator.

b.   Verifying that the investigator has adequate qualifications and resources (see 4.1,4.2,5.6) which remain adequate throughout the trial period, that facilities, including laboratories, equipment, and staff, are adequate to safely and properly conduct the trial and remain adequate throughout the trial period.

d.   Verifying that the investigator follows the approved protocol and all approved amendment(s), if any.

g.   Ensuring that the investigator and the investigator's staff are adequately informed about the trial.

k.   Verifying that source documents and other trial records are accurate, complete, kept up-to-date and maintained.

m.   Checking the accuracy and completeness of the CRF entries, source documents and other trial-related records against each other. The monitor specifically should verify that:

i.   The data required by the protocol are reported accurately on the CRFs and are consistent with the source documents.

ii.   Any dose and/or therapy modifications are well documented for each of the trial subjects.

284   The Survive and Thrive Guide to Computer Validation

> iii.   Adverse events, concomitant medications and intercurrent illnesses are reported in accordance with the protocol on the CRFs.
>
> iv.   Visits that the subjects fail to make, tests that are not conducted, and examinations that are not performed are clearly reported as such on the CRFs.
>
> v.   All withdrawals and dropouts of enrolled subjects from the trial are reported and explained on the CRFs.

n.   Informing the investigator of any CRF entry error, omission, or illegibility. The monitor should ensure that appropriate corrections, additions, or deletions are made, dated, explained (if necessary), and initialed by the investigator or by a member of the investigator's trial staff who is authorized to initial CRF changes for the investigator. This authorization should be documented.

ICH and FDA Guidelines for GCP Systems—Excerpts

FDA Draft Guidance—
Computerized Systems Used in Clinical Trials

This guidance document is being distributed for comment purposes only. Draft released for comment on June 18, 1997. Draft—Not for Implementation.

I. Introduction

This document addresses issues pertaining to computer systems used to generate, collect, maintain, and transmit clinical data intended for submission to the Food and Drug Administration (FDA) in support of marketing or research applications. These data form the basis for the Agency's decisions regarding the safety and effectiveness of new human and animal drugs, biologicals, medical devices, and certain food and color additives. As such, these data have broad public health significance and must be of the highest quality and integrity.

FDA established the Bioresearch Monitoring (BIMO) Program of inspections and audits to monitor the conduct and reporting of clinical trials to ensure that data meet the highest standards of quality and integrity and conform to FDA's regulations for clinical trials. FDA's acceptance of data from clinical trials for decision-making purposes is dependent upon its ability to validate the quality and integrity of such data during its onsite inspections and audits. To be acceptable, the data should meet certain fundamental elements of quality whether collected or recorded electronically or on paper. Data should be attributable, original, accurate, contemporaneous and legible. For example, attributable data can be traced to the individual responsible for observing and recording the data. In an automated system, such an element could be addressed by a computer system designed to record the identity of the individual responsible for any input.

The guidance offered in this document is intended to address how these elements of data quality might be satisfied in a clinical environment where computerized systems are being used to generate, record, and maintain data. Persons using the data from computerized systems should have confidence that the data are at least as reliable as data in paper form.

This guidance has been prepared by an Agency working group representing the Bioresearch Monitoring Program Managers from each Center within FDA and the Office of Regulatory Affairs. As with other guidance documents, the FDA does not intend this guidance document to be all-inclusive and cautions that not all information will apply to all situations.

286   The Survive and Thrive Guide to Computer Validation

This guidance should not supplant discussions between Centers and sponsors regarding format and content of electronic applications before the submission of marketing or research applications or before the initiation of trials. Modifications may be necessary for specific protocols. Due to the unique nature of clinical trials, FDA Centers have the responsibility to determine the acceptability of a protocol.

II.   Definitions

Audit Trail is a secure time stamped record that allows reconstruction of the course of events relating to the creation, modification, and deletion of an electronic study record.

Certified Copy is a copy of original information that has been verified, as indicated by dated signature, as an exact copy having all of the same attributes and information as the original.

Commit means a saving action that creates or modifies, or an action that deletes, an electronic record or portion of an electronic record. For example, pressing the "Enter" key of a keyboard after information is typed to enter the information into the record.

Computerized System includes computer hardware, software, and associated documents that generate, collect, maintain, or transmit in digital form information related to the conduct of a clinical trial.

Direct Entry means recording of data where an electronic record is the original capture of the data. Examples are the keying by an individual of original observations into the system, or automatic recording by the system of the output of a balance that measures subjects' body weight. Electronic Case Report Form (e-CRF) is an auditable permanent electronic record designed to record all of the protocol required information to be reported to the sponsor on each trial subject.

Electronic Patient Diary is an electronic record into which a subject participating in a clinical trial directly enters observations or directly responds to an evaluation checklist.

Electronic Record is any combination of text, graphics, data, audio, pictorial, or any other information representation in digital form that is created, modified, maintained, archived, retrieved, or distributed by a computer system.

Electronic Signature is a computer data compilation of any symbol or series of symbols, executed, adopted, or authorized by an individual to be the legally binding equivalent of the individual's handwritten signature.

ICH and FDA Guidelines for GCP Systems—Excerpts   287

Source Data is all information in original records and certified copies of original records of clinical findings, observations, or other activities in a clinical trial necessary for the reconstruction and evaluation of the trial. Source data are contained in source documents (original records or certified copies).

Source Documents are original documents and records including, but not limited to, hospital records, clinical and office charts, laboratory notes, memoranda, subjects' diaries or evaluation checklists, pharmacy dispensing records, recorded data from automated instruments, copies or transcriptions certified after verification as being accurate and complete, microfiches, photographic negatives, microfilm or magnetic media, x-rays, subject files, and records kept at the pharmacy, at the laboratories, and at medico-technical departments involved in the clinical trial.

III. *General Principles*

A. When original observations are entered directly into a computer system, the electronic record is the source data.

B. A computerized system should ensure that all applicable regulatory requirements for record keeping and record retention in clinical trials are met with at least the same degree of confidence as is provided with paper systems.

C. Clinical investigators should retain copies of all records and underlying data sent to a sponsor or contract research organization including query resolution correspondence.

D. Any correction to a record required to be maintained should not obscure the original entry; this applies to both written and electronic corrections.

E. Changes to data that are stored on electronic media will always require an audit trail, per 21 CFR 11.10(e). For changes made at the research site, the clinical investigator's documentation should include who made the changes, and when, how, and why they were made.

F. The FDA may audit any and all records that might support submissions to the Agency, regardless of how they were created or maintained.

G. Data should be retrievable in such a fashion that all information regarding each individual subject in a study is attributable to that subject.

H. A computerized system should be designed so that all requirements outlined in a study protocol are satisfied (e.g., upper or lower limits for laboratory analyses, requirements that the study be blinded) and so that requirements for the preparation and maintenance of case histories are not adversely affected by creation or storage by electronic means.

288   The Survive and Thrive Guide to Computer Validation

I.   Study protocols should state which computerized systems are to be used for generation, collection, maintenance, and transmission of data.

J.   Security measures should be in place to prevent unauthorized access to the data and the data collection device.

IV.   Standard Operating Procedures

Standard operating procedures (SOPs) pertinent to the use of the computerized system should be available at the clinical site.

SOPs should be established for, but not limited to:

- System Setup/Installation
- Data Collection
- System Maintenance
- Data Backup and Recovery
- Security
- Change Control

V.   Data Entry

A.   Electronic Signatures

1.   The data entry system should be designed so that individuals need to enter electronic signatures, such as combined password/usernames or biometric-based electronic signatures, before entering information for a given data entry session.

2.   Each entry to an electronic record, including any change, should be made under the electronic signature of the individual making that entry.

   a.   In systems where an individual is entering data directly, the printed name of that individual should be visible on the data entry screen throughout the data entry session. This is intended to preclude the possibility of a different individual inadvertently entering data under someone else's name.

   b.   If the name displayed on the screen during a data entry session is not that of the person entering the data, then that individual should log on under his or her own name before continuing.

3. Passwords should not be shared among individuals

4. Passwords should be changed at regular intervals.

ICH and FDA Guidelines for GCP Systems—Excerpts   289

5.   When someone leaves a workstation, the person should log off the system. Failing this, an automatic log off may be appropriate for long idle periods. For short periods of inactivity, an automatic screen saver with password could be coupled with a locked keypad or pointing device.

B.   Audit Trails

1.   21 CFR 11.10(e) requires persons who use electronic record systems to maintain an audit trail to protect the authenticity, integrity, and, when appropriate, the confidentiality of electronic records. According to the regulation:

    a.   Persons must use secure, computer-generated, time-stamped audit trails to independently record the date and time of operator entries and actions that create, modify, or delete electronic records.

    b.   Record changes must not obscure previously recorded information.

    c.   Audit trail documentation must be retained for a period at least as long as that required for the subject electronic records (e.g., the study data and records to which they pertain) and must be available for agency review and copying.

2.   Personnel who create, modify, or delete electronic records should not be able to modify the audit trails.

3.   Audit trails in computer-assisted clinical trials should be retained as part of the basic electronic study records.

4.   Audit trail files should be retained wherever the records covered by the audit trails are maintained.

5.   Audit trail files should be created incrementally, in chronological order, and in a manner that does not allow new audit trail information to overwrite existing data in violation of §11.10(e).

C.   Date/Time Stamps

1.   Controls should be in place to ensure that, upon each boot-up, the system's date and time are correct and that the date and time are not changed by unauthorized means.

2.   The system's date and time should be used to generate the date and time applied to audit trails and records.

3.   Dates and times should be local to the activity being documented and should include the year, month, day, hour, and minute. The Agency encourages establishments to synchronize systems to the date and time

290   The Survive and Thrive Guide to Computer Validation

provided by trusted third parties. Clinical study data collection devices will likely be used in multi-center trials, perhaps located in different time zones. When a data-handling device is transported to the site of use, it is important that its time be checked and correctly set to local time.

The ability to change the date or time should be limited to authorized personnel and such personnel should be notified if a system date or time discrepancy is detected. Changes to date or time should be documented.

VI. *System Design*

A.   Systems used for direct entry of data should include features that will facilitate the collection of quality data.

   1.   Prompts, flags or help features within the data collection device should be used to ensure that clinical terminology or adverse event terms are consistent with the specific study protocol. Such features should also alert the user to data that are out of acceptable range.

   2.   Electronic patient diaries and electronic case report forms (e-CRFs) should be designed to allow users to make annotations. Annotations add to data quality by allowing ad hoc information to be captured. This information may be valuable in the event of an adverse reaction or outlier. The record should clearly indicate who recorded the annotations and when (date and time).

B.   Systems used for direct entry of data should be designed to include features that will facilitate the inspection and review of data.

Data tags (e.g., different color, different font, flags) should be used to indicate which data have been changed or deleted.

C.   Recognizing that computer products may be discontinued, sponsors should make certain that continued support for the automated system is available to ensure data integrity is maintained over the life of the study, and as necessary for record retrieval and review. Such support should cover all versions of application software, operating systems, compilers, linkers, and other development tools involved in processing data or records.

VII. *Security*

A.   **Physical Security**

1.   In addition to internal safeguards built into the system, external safeguards should be in place to ensure that access to the data collection device and to the data is restricted to authorized, trained personnel.

ICH and FDA Guidelines for GCP Systems—Excerpts 291

2. Staff should be thoroughly aware of system security measures and the importance of limiting access to authorized personnel.

3. Names of authorized staff members, their titles, and a description of their access privileges should be in the study documentation.

4. SOPs should be in place for handling and storing the system to prevent unauthorized access.

5. External safeguards should include lock-and-key storage of the data and collection devices.

B. Logical Security

1. Access to the database at the clinical site should be restricted through the system's software with its required log-on, security procedures, and audit trail. The data should not be altered, browsed, queried, or reported via external software applications that do not enter through the protective system software.

2. If a sponsor or contract research organization supplies a computerized system exclusively for a clinical trial, the system should remain dedicated to the purpose for which it was intended and validated.

3. If a computerized system being used for the clinical study is part of the system normally used by the practitioner, efforts should be made to ensure that the software is logically and physically isolated as necessary to preclude unintended interaction with non-study software. The system should be reevaluated if any of the software programs are changed.

VIII. System Dependability

A. Documentation should be readily available at the site where clinical trials are conducted, to provide an overall description of computerized operations and the relationship of hardware, software, and physical environment in these computerized operations.

B. The sponsor should ensure and document that the electronic data processing system conforms to the sponsor's established requirements for completeness, accuracy, reliability, and consistent performance for the intended purpose.

C. The FDA inspects documentation, possessed by a regulated company, that demonstrates validation of software. The study sponsor is responsible for making such documentation available for inspection at the study site if requested. Clinical investigators are not generally responsible for validation unless they originated or modified software.

292 The Survive and Thrive Guide to Computer Validation

1. In the case of software purchased off-the-shelf, most of the validation should have been done by the company that wrote the software. The sponsor or contract research organization should have documentation of this design level validation by the vendor, and should have itself performed functional testing (e.g., by use of test data sets).

   In the special case of database and spreadsheet software (1) that is purchased off-the-shelf, (2) that is designed for and widely used for general purposes, (3) is unmodified, and (4) is not being used for direct entry of data, the sponsor or contract research organization may not have documentation of design level validation. However, the sponsor or contract research organization itself should have performed functional testing (e.g., by use of test data sets) and researched known software limitations, problems, and defect corrections.

2. Documentation important to demonstrate software validation should include:

   a. Written design specification that describes what the software is intended to do and how it is intended to do it.

   b. A written test plan based on the design specification, including both structural and functional analysis.

   c. Test results and an evaluation of how these results demonstrate that the predetermined criteria have been met.

D. Change Control

1. Written procedures should be in place to ensure that changes to the computerized system such as software upgrades, equipment or component replacement, or new instrumentation will not jeopardize the integrity of the data or the integrity of protocols.

2. All changes to the system should be documented. Changes that exceed operational limits or design specifications should precipitate revalidation.

IX. System Controls

A. Software Version Control

Measures should be in place to ensure that versions of software used to generate, collect, maintain, and transmit data are the versions that are stated in the systems documentation.

B. Contingency Plans

Written procedures should describe contingency plans for conducting the study by alternate means in the event of failure of the computerized system.

C. Backup and Recovery

1.   Backup and recovery procedures should be clearly outlined in the standard operating procedures and be sufficient to protect against data loss. Data should be backed up regularly in a way that would prevent a catastrophic loss.

2.   Backup data should be stored at a secure location specified in the SOP and separate from the original records. This should include offsite storage.

3.   Backup and recovery operations should be documented to permit an assessment of the nature and scope of possible data loss resulting from a system failure.

X.   *Training of Personnel*

A. Qualifications

1.   Each person who enters or processes data should have the education, training, and experience or any combination thereof necessary to perform the assigned functions.

2.   Individuals responsible for monitoring the trial should have education, training, and experience in the use of the computerized system necessary to adequately monitor the trial.

B. Training

1.   Training should be provided to individuals in the specific operations that they are to perform.

2.   Training should be conducted by qualified individuals on a continuing basis, as needed, to ensure familiarity with the computerized system and with any changes to the system during the course of the study.

3.   Training should include but is not limited to:

- •   System setup/installation
- •   Instruction in the proper use of equipment
- •   Data collection

294   The Survive and Thrive Guide to Computer Validation

- • System maintenance
- • Backup and recovery
- • Security measures

C.   Documentation

Employee qualifications, training and experience should be documented.

XI.   Records Inspection

A.   The FDA may audit any and all records that might support submissions to the Agency, regardless of how they were created or maintained. Therefore, systems should be able to generate accurate and complete copies of records in both human readable and electronic form suitable for inspection, review, and copying by the Agency. Persons should contact the appropriate Agency unit if there is any doubt about what file formats and media the Agency can read and copy.

B.   The sponsor should be able to provide hardware and software as necessary for FDA personnel to inspect the electronic documents and audit trail at the site where an FDA inspection is taking place.

XII.   Certification of Electronic Signatures

When electronic signatures are used to meet an FDA signature requirement, persons using the system must submit a certification to the agency that the persons intend their electronic signatures to be legally binding, per 21 CFR §11.100(c).

As set forth in 21 CFR 11.100(c), the certification is to be submitted in paper form signed with a traditional handwritten signature to the Office of Regional Operations (HFC-100), 5600 Fishers Lane, Rockville Maryland 20857. The certification is to be submitted prior to or at the time electronic signatures are used. However, a single certification may cover all electronic signatures used by persons in a given organization. An acceptable certification would take the following format:

Pursuant to Section 11.100 of Title 21 of the Code of Federal Regulations, this is to certify that [name of organization] intends that all electronic signatures executed by our employees, agents, or representatives, located anywhere in the world, are the legally binding equivalent of traditional handwritten signatures.

This "certification" is a legal document created by persons to acknowledge that their electronic signatures have the same legal significance as their traditional handwritten signatures.

XIII. References

FDA, *Software Development Activities*, 1987.

FDA, *Guideline for the Monitoring of Clinical Investigations*, 1988.

FDA, *Conduct of Clinical Investigations: Responsibilities of Clinical Investigators and Monitors for Investigational New Animal Drug Studies*, 1992.

FDA, *Compliance Program Guidance Manual*, "Compliance Program 7348.810—Sponsors, Contract Research Organizations and Monitors," August 18, 1994.

FDA, *Compliance Program Guidance Manual*, "Compliance Program 7348.811—Bioresearch Monitoring—Clinical Investigations," August 18, 1994.

FDA, *Information Sheets for Institutional Review Boards and Clinical Investigators*, 1995.

FDA, *Glossary of Computerized System and Software Development Terminology*, 1995.

Organisation for Economic Cooperation and Development (OECD), *The Application of the Principles of GLP to Computerised Systems*, Environmental Monograph No. 116, Paris, 1995.

International Conference on Harmonisation; "Good Clinical Practice: Consolidated Guideline" *Federal Register*, Vol. 62, No. 90, 25711, May 9, 1997.

FDA, "21 CFR Part 11, Electronic Records; Electronic Signatures; Final Rule." *Federal Register*, Vol. 62, No. 54, 13429, March 20, 1997.

Index

Acceptance
    criteria, 268
    testing, 45, 70–71, 268
Access control, in operations phase of system life
    cycle, 29–30
Acquisition process, 22–23
Annex 11. *See* GMP Guide Annex 11
Archives, 195–197
Audit Reports
    legacy system and, 93
    retrospective work and, 80, 83–84
Audits/inspections
    automation logbook and, 192, 197–198
    definitions, 279, 286
    e-data compliance and, 203
    EDQ Plan Checklist and, 209
    general checklist for, 181–182
    GMP manufacturing systems and, 220
    in system owner's validation package, 58, 62
    laboratory systems, 196–198
    logs, 115, 179–180
    objective of, 166–167
    of supplier's Quality Plan, 48–49
    personnel preparation for, 232–233
    QA and, 48–49
    reports of validation package, 74–75
    SOPs for, 169, 173, 176–179
    SQAP and, 114–115
    system owner's validation role in, 58, 62, 78
    validation documentation and, 30, 74–75
    vendor, 120

Backup/recovery, 9–10, 268
Biometrics, 149
Black box testing, 29, 93
    GALP laboratory regulations and, 190
    SQAP, 115–117
Blue Book. *See* FDA Blue Book
Branch testing, 115
Branning, R.C., 71
Budgeting
    reasons for validation, 12–13, 58–59
    role of system sponsor in, 2–4
    system owner's validation package and, 58

Business applications. *See* Budgeting; Operating
    environment

Case Report Form (CRF), 279
Certified copy, 286
cGMP (current Good Manufacturing Practices).
    See GMP
Change control, 268
    "novel elements" and, 226–227
    configuration management and, 45
    FDA Blue Book inspections and, 153
    GALP laboratory regulations and, 188, 192
    GMP manufacturing systems and, 220
    in operations phase of system life cycle, 29–30
    log, 45, 88–89
    quality assurance of, 9–10
Chapman, K.G., 71
Chromatography, 183–184
Clinical research organizations (CROs), 200–201
Clinical research systems, 199–203
Closed system, 149–151
C.M. Logbook, 119, 122
COA (Certificate of Analysis), 222, 229
Coding
    as found in engineering SOPs, 44–45
    logical security and, 12
    management system of, 45–46
    media control, 122
    programming and configuring, 25–26
    source, 269
    Validation Plan and, 118–119
Combination testing, 115–117
Commission, SDLC and, 27–29
Commission Phase Testing, 70–71
Computerized systems, 268, 286
    clinical research and, 199
    EU GMP Guide Annex 11, 165–166
    FDA Blue Book regulations and, 143
    GLP C.V. Policy, 125–127
    GMP manufacturing systems, 217–218
    inspection standards, 169
    integrity of, 180–181
    IT (information technology) as, 15–16
    laboratory management (LIMS), 183–188

297

298 The Survive and Thrive Guide to Computer Validation

MHW GMP Guideline, 155, 157–160
OECD GLP Consensus for, 73, 147–148, 150–152
protocol-specific, 205–207
reliability factors of, 214
retirement of, 195
SQAP and, 106–108, 115–118
Computer systems, 219–220, 268
  concepts and components, 5–9
  definition, 286
  documentation of verification for, 50–51
  FDA Blue Book inspections and, 153–154
  FDA inspection and regulation of e-records, 149, 151
  OECD GLP Consensus Document, 73
  regulations of closed and open, 149–151
  URS components, 20
  validation life cycle phases/activities, 15–17, 133–134
  Validation Test Plan, 64–65, 78
Computer Systems Validation Committee (CSVC), computer system concepts of, 5
Computer Validation Policy. See C.V. Policy,
Computer validation. See Validation
Configuration management
  EDQ Plan and, 211, 213–214
  logs for, 42
  SQAP problem reporting, 116, 118
Contractors, 223–224
Corrective action, 116, 118–119. See also Problems
CRAs (clinical research associates), 209–214
CRFs (case report forms), electronic, 200, 205–206
C.V. Policy
  as audit and review standards, 169, 173
  business benefits of, 140–141
  development and contents of, 127–132
  documentation model for, 133, 137–138
  GALP laboratory regulations and, 191
  GMP manufacturing systems and, 223–225
  inspection response model for, 133, 139–140
  integration of regulations via, 102–104
  management model for, 133, 135–136
  role for senior management in, 125–127
  SOPs and, 126–127
  SQAP and, 135–140
  standard system model for, 133, 138–139
  system life cycle model, 133–135
  trial sponsor systems and, 201, 203
  use of directives for GXP systems in, 162–163

Data
  audit/inspection of, 182
  collection process using ICH GCP, 161–162
  EDQ Plan, 208–209, 213
  electronic records retention, 195–196
  for tests, 52–53
  found in engineering SOPs, 43–45

  GALP handling of, 183–186, 188, 190–192
  GCP system, 201–202, 215
  handling in Transition Plan, 33–34
  ICH GCP validation of e-records, 159, 161
  inclusion in Needs Analysis, 17–18
  inclusion in RFP, 19
  inclusion in validation testing, 66–68, 72
  input via PC and WAN, 8
  in retrospective evaluation package, 80
  QA and, 207, 215
  raw, 196–197, 205–206
  remote entry systems, 204–206
  source, 280, 287
  storage and retrieval of electronic, 148, 150–152
Data integrity, 59, 180–181, 185–186, 202–203, 209
  electronic records and signatures, 230–232
  GMP manufacturing systems and, 220
Data Managment Plan, 201, 205, 207
DCS, 220, 224
Decommission of validated system, 31–34. See also Retirement
Design of system. See SDD
Desk test (QC), 93, 96
Development documentation, 47–48
Device GMP, 154–156, 163
Digital signature, 150
Direct entry, 286
Directives. See Regulations; Standards; specific titles
Disaster recovery
  code and media control SOPs, 119, 122
  management responsibilities, 127, 182
Documentation. See also Logs
  audit/inspection checklist, 181–182
  automation logbook and, 192, 197–198
  C.V. Policy and, 133, 137–138
  definition, 279–280
  development during SDLC, 47–48
  FDA Blue Book inspections and, 153–154
  FDA inspection and regulation of e-records, 149–152
  for "novel elements," 227
  for supplier's SDLC QA, 42
  importance in retrospective work, 83–85
  in operations phase of system life cycle, 29–30
  legacy system and, 194–196
  manufacturing system SOPs, 224–227
  of configuration management, 71–72
  of software testing in clinical research, 203
  SQAP, 111, 124
  system, 2
  system owner's validation testing, 66
  tests and test plans, 51–55
Documents
  contacts for acquiring, 235–236, 257
  FDA regulations, 143–144, 149–152

Index   299

in retrospective evaluation package, 80
OECD GLP Consensus, 73, 147–148, 150–152
retrospective system and user, 91–92
source, 280, 287
SQAP reference, 109
supplier's verification testing and inclusion of, 50–51
system and user, 75–76
use of encryption in, 231
user requirements, 92
Drug GMP
documentation and enforcement, 252
objectives, 243
operation control, 248–251
system development, 244–248

e-data. *See* Electronic records; Electronic signatures
EDQ (e-Data Quality) Plan, 207–212
Electromagnetic interference (EMI), 155
Electronic CRFs, 200, 205–206
Electronic points, 191–192
Electronic records
data integrity of, 208, 212–214
definition, 286
diaries, 204, 204, 286
FDA 21 CFR Part 11, 149–152, 253–254, 268
FDA Final Rule inspection of, 169–171
laboratory systems and, 195–197
manufacturing systems and, 230–232
SOPs and, 196–197, 203, 209, 231–232
Electronic signatures, 163
data integrity of, 208, 212–214
definition, 268, 286
FDA 21 CFR Part 11, 149–152, 255–256, 268, 288–289
FDA Draft Guidelines, 288–289
FDA Final Rule inspection of, 169–171
manufacturing systems and, 230–232
SQAP and, 122–123
Electrostatic discharge (ESD), 155
Encryption use, 231
Engineering SOPs, 43–45, 47–48
Environmental system control, 155
EPA
2185 Good Automated Laboratory Practices (GALP), 184–186, 270–275
document contacts, 257
e-Quality/e-Q, 207
EU document contacts, 235
EU GMP Guide Annex 11, 162. *See also* GMP; OECD GLP Consensus
computerized systems, 237–239
computerized systems life cycle, 133–134
contract manufacture and analysis (Chapter 7), 240–243

documentation (Chapter 4), 239–240
GMP manufacturing systems and, 218–220
inspections, 165–166
laboratories and, 186
manufacturing systems and, 226
requirements for computerized systems, 145–146, 150–152
EU GMP. *See* GMP
European Agency for the Evaluation of Medicinal Products (EMEA)
ICH GCP validation and, 159, 161
OECD GLP Consensus and, 73, 147–148, 150–152
European Union. *See* EU
Evaluation. *See* Testing
Evaluation Summary Report
retrospective, 97–98
sponsor role in, 79–80
Evaluation testing, 94–96

FDA
electronic records document 21 CFR Part 11, 144
Form 483 audit report, 179
GCP document sources, 277–278
regulations, 143–144
FDA 21 CFR Part 11
electronic records, 253–254
electronic records and signatures, 149–152, 230–232
electronic signatures, 255–256
Final Rule, 149–152, 169–171
FDA Blue Book, 152–154, 163
validation regulations, 143
FDA Draft Guidance, 285–294
data entry, 288–290
definitions, 286–287
document contacts, 236
electronic signature certification, 294
general principles, 287–288
introduction, 285–286
records inspection, 294
security, 290–291
SOPs, 288
system controls, 292–293
system dependability, 291–292
system design, 290
training of personnel, 293–294
Final Rule. *See* FDA
Full-system testing, 45
Functional testing, 115–117
Funding. *See* Budgeting

GALP (Good Automated Laboratory Practices), 184–191, 270–275
Gap analysis
GALP laboratory regulations and, 186

300   The Survive and Thrive Guide to Computer Validation

of GMP manufacturing systems, 221
walk-through review and, 174–175
GC/LC. *See* Chromatography
GCP (Good Clinical Practices) *See also* GXP
action for violation of, 180
definition, 280
document sources, 277
inclusion in Needs Analysis Report, 18
reliability factors, 214
SQAP and, 103
system QA
validation of specialty systems, 204, 215
General operating procedures (GOPs). *See* GOPs
GLP Consensus Document
application of GLP principles to computerized
systems, 259–268
approach, 258–259
legacy automation system and, 194–196
retrospective evaluation and, 86–88
scope, 258
GLP. *See also* GXP; OECD GLP
action for violation of, 180
application to computerized systems, 73,
147–148, 150–152
inclusion in Needs Analysis Report, 18
OECD and, 144–145, 150–152
OECD C.V. Policy and, 125–127
SQAP and, 103
GMP for Bulk Drug Substances. *See* Drug GMP
GMP for Pharmaceutical Products (MHW Ordinance No. 31). *See* Drug GMP
GMP Guide Annex 11. *See also* OECD GLP Consensus
computerized systems, 237–239
computerized systems life cycle, 133–134
contract manufacture and analysis (Chapter 7),
240–243
documentation (Chapter 4), 239–240
requirements for computerized systems,
145–146, 150–152
GMP. *See also* GXP
action for violation of, 180
FDA regulations of, 144
inclusion in Needs Analysis Report, 18
manufacturing systems and, 217–218, 222–
227, 233
medical device application and, 154–155
personnel knowledge of, 228
SQAP and, 103, 117–118, 226, 233
Good Automated Laboratory Practices. *See* GALP;
GLP
Good Clinical Practice. *See* GCP
*Good Computer Validation Practices: Common Sense
Implementation*
Good Laboratory Practices. *See* GLP

Good Manufacturing Practice. *See* Drug GMP; EU
GMP; GMP
GOPs, 113–114, 120
Gray box testing, 115–117
*Guideline on Control of Computerized Systems in
Drug Manufacturing*, 155, 157–160
*Guide to Inspection of Computerized Systems in Drug
Processing*, 143
GXP (Good X Practices)
computer validation matrix and, 132
C.V. Directives for, 162–163
C.V. Policy and, 126–127, 130–132
inclusion in Needs Analysis Report, 18
validation for software acquisition, 20, 22–23

Hardware
definition, 268
environmental control for, 155
FDA Blue Book inspections and, 153–154
PLCs, 8–9
SQAP testing and, 117
Help (online). *See also* Training materials, 9–11
History of system, 81, 83–85

ICH Draft Guideline on Statistical Principles
for clinical trials, 202–203, 215
GCP and, 161, 163
ICH GCP. *See also* GXP, 144–145, 163
clinical research systems and, 200
data collection process and, 161–162
Directive, 159, 161
ICH GCP Topic E6, 279–284
definitions, 279–280
introduction, 279
investigator's responsibilities, 281
monitor's responsibilities, 283–284
principles of, 280–281
sponsor's responsibilities, 281–284
IEEE Std. 1012–1986
software verification and validation, 81–82
software verification and validation plans, 43–44
Validation Plan outline, 61–63
IEEE Std. 1012-1987, software verification and validation plans, 77–78
IEEE Std. 1016.1-1993, SDD and, 47
IEEE Std. 1016-1987, SDD and, 47
IEEE Std. 1062-1993, software acquisition, 20,
22–23
IEEE Std. 610.12-1990, software engineering terminology, 51–52
IEEE Std. 730-1989, software QA plans, 104–105
IEEE Std. 829-1983, software test documentation,
95, 65, 67
IEEE Std. Glossary of Software Engineering Ter-
minology, 166–167

Index   301

Inspection Response Team. *See* IRT
Inspections. *See also* Audits/inspections
    FDA Blue Book and, 152–154
    importance of validation documentation, 30
    objective of, 166–167
    personnel preparation for, 232–233
    preapproval, 168
    response model, 133, 139–140
    SOPs for, 176–179
    unannounced FDA, 168–169
    validation risk and, 122
Installation and operation, 158–159
Installation Qualification. *See* IQ
Institute for Electrical and Electronic Engineers,
    Inc. *See* IEEE
Instruction manuals. *See* Training materials
Integration testing, 26, 45
Interface testing, 45
Internal service level agreement (ISLA), 74
International clinical studies, 206–207
International Conference on Harmonization. *See*
    ICH GCP
International Organization for Standardization.
    See ISO
International regulations and standards. *See also*
    IEEE; ISO
    System sponsor and, 143–145
    use of directives for GXP systems, 162–163
Inventory, GALP laboratory regulations and, 186
IQ (Installation Qualification)
    of qualification testing, 71
    of SQAP, 116–117
    system acceptance and, 27
IRT (inspection response team). *See also* Inspections
    inspection response model and, 115, 167–168
    model, 140, 167–168
    walk-through review and, 172–176
ISO 9000, inclusion in Needs Analysis Report, 18
ISO 9000-3, 39–41
    contract items on quality, 20–21
    Final Rule, 169
    supplier management and, 120–121
IT (information technology), 15–16

Laboratory Information Management System. *See*
    LIMS
Laboratory system e-records, 195–197
Ladder logic, 8–9
Language, in SOPs, 43
LC. *See* Chromatography
Legacy systems
    automation of, 193–195
    documentation of, 83
    evaluation testing of, 94–96
    OECD GLP Consensus and, 73, 147–148

product life cycle and, 228–230
retrospective evaluation package and, 79, 98–99
Life cycle
    acquisition process, 22–23
    computer validation of, 133–134
    GALP laboratory regulations and, 189–190
    phases/activities, 15–17
LIMS raw data (LRD)
    definition, 275
    GALP and, 183–188
    legacy automation system and, 193–194
    use of data handling model in, 190–192
Logical security. *See also* Security
    quality assurance of, 9, 11–12
    retrospective work and, 84
    validation risk and, 122
Logs
    audit, 115
    Audit/Inspection Report, 179–180
    configuration management, 45–46
    in operations phase of system life cycle, 29–30
    instrument automation, 192
    in supplier's verification package, 38
    in system owner's validation package, 58, 62
    result, 52–53, 66–67
    retest, 88, 90
    retrospective work and, 83–84, 86
    standard system validation package, 139
    supplier's SDLC QA and, 42
    support and service in configuration manage-
      ment, 46
    system management, 74–75, 88–91
LRD. *See* LIMS raw data

Maintenance
    audit/Inspection and, 182
    instrument automation logbook and, 192
    in system life cycle, 30–31
    system life cycle phases/activities, 16–17
    system owner's validation role in, 58, 62
Management
    control, 2
    C.V. Policy and, 133, 135–136
    GMP manufacturing systems and, 220
    laboratory (LIMS), 183–188
    role in C.V. Policy, 125–129
    SQAP development and, 107, 109–111
    system sponsor, 1–2
Manufacturing operating environment. *See* Oper-
    ating environment
Manufacturing systems, 217–220
Media control in Validation Plan, 119
Medical device GMP, 154–156
Medical Device GMP Manual, 154–155
Medical Monitoring Plan, 201, 205, 207

302　The Survive and Thrive Guide to Computer Validation

MHW (Japan)
　document contacts, 235
　drug manufacturing guidelines (Drug GMP),
　　243–252
　GMP Guideline for computerized systems,
　　155–160, 163
　OECD GLP Consensus and, 73, 147–148,
　　150–152
MHW Ordinance No. 31. *See* Drug GMP
Ministry of Health and Welfare (Japan). *See* MHW
　(Japan)
Monitoring, 280
MRPs (materials resource planning systems), 103
Multiple systems, 102–103

Needs Analysis
　in validation package, 58, 62, 139
　making a report, 17–18
　need for Transition Plan included in, 32
　QA and, 18
　system life cycle phases/activities, 15–17
Needs Analysis Report
　legacy system and, 92
　supplier control and, 120
Network security, quality assurance of, 9, 11–12.
　See also Security
New Drug Application (NDA), 228–229
Nonsponsor systems, 201–203, 214–215

Observations, original, 275
OECD GLP, 144–145
　Consensus Document, 73, 147–148, 150–
　　152, 162
　C.V. Policy and, 125–127
　document contacts, 257
　laboratories and, 186
　legacy automation system and system retire-
　　ment, 194–196
　legacy system and, 87–88, 92
　retrospective evaluation and, 86–88
Online help. *See also* Training materials, 9–11
Open system e-records, 149–151
Operational Qualification. *See* OQ
Operation Phase Validation, 71–72
Operations
　phase of system life cycle, 29–30
　system documents of, 50–51
　system life cycle phases/activities, 16–17
　system owner's validation role in, 58, 62
OQ (Operational Qualification)
　of qualification testing, 71
　of SQAP, 116–117
　system acceptance and, 27
Organization for Economic Cooperation and De-
　velopment. *See* OECD

Original Medical Record. *See* Source documents
Original observations, 275
Owner. *See* System owner
Owner's Validation Package, 57–59

PAB Natification No. 598. *See* Drug GMP
Passwords, 12
Path testing, 115
Peer review (SDLC), 26
Performance Qualification (PQ). *See* PQ
Peripheral components, 268
Personal codes, logical security and, 12
Personnel
　for verification activities, 39–40
　preparation for audits/inspections, 232–233
　safety in manufacturing systems and, 217–218
　training to GMP validation, 227–228
Physical security. *See also* Security
　quality assurance of, 9, 11–12
　retrospective work and, 84
　validation risk and, 122
Platform supplier, as member of system team, 3–4
Platform support
　in system owner's validation package, 58, 62
　of validation package, 74
Platform system
　of operating environment, 7–9
　retrospective work and, 84
　SQAP testing and, 117
PLC (programmable logic controllers), 8–9, 220
PMA model, 6–7
Policy Team. *See* C.V. Policy
PQ (Performance Qualification), 71, 116
Preapproval inspections, 168
Priorities, in validation of GMP systems, 217–219
Problems. *See also* Change control; SEQ
　inclusion of "novel elements," 226–227
　in operations phase of system life cycle, 29–30
　lack of retrospective documentation, 91–92
　logs for, 46
　product and personnel safety, 217–218
　reporting of, 116, 118, 182
　resolution of, 51
Process system. *See also* Computerized system, 5
Proposal. *See* Request for proposal (RFP)
Protocol. *See* Trial sponsor systems
Protocol-specific systems, 205–207
Purchaser of system, 40–42, 121

QA (quality assurance). *See also* SQAP
　audit reports and, 74–75
　backup/recovery, 9–10, 268
　GMP manufacturing system software, 220
　help systems, 9–11
　inclusion in Needs Analysis Report, 18

inspection response model and, 140, 167–168
of e-data and e-systems, 207, 215
roles in SQAP, 4, 110, 112
SCADA and, 8–9
software, 114–115, 117
standard system model for, 9–11
supplier of system and, 42
supplier Self-Audit Reports and, 48–49
validation package and, 58–59, 62
validations in operations phase of system life
cycle and, 30
walk-through review and, 172–176
QC (quality control)
as member of system team, 4
desk test of, 93
GALP laboratory regulations and, 190
in operations phase of system life cycle, 29–30
legacy system and, 93
of validation package, 75, 78
retrospective evaluation and, 81–83
roles in SQAP, 110, 112
Qualification testing, 70–71

Raw data, 196–197, 205–206
RDE (remote data entry), 205–206
Recognized technical standards (definition), 268
Record protection. *See* Security
Records
archiving and retention in laboratory systems,
195–197
electronic, 149–152, 230–232, 253–254, 268
management, 120–121
retrospective work and, 83–84
system managment logs, 88–91
Recovery. *See* Disaster recovery
Regulations. *See also specific names*; Standards
EPA GALP laboratory, 184–186
FDA Blue Book, 143, 152–154, 163
MHW (Japan), 73, 147–152, 155–160, 235,
243–252
OECD C.V. Policy, 125–127
SQAP development and, 107
timeline, 143–144
Reliability of system, 2
Replacement of validated system, 31–34
Replication
contract items on quality (ISO 9000-3), 21
requirements of, 121
Reports. *See also* Logs; Records
audit/inspection, 179–180
evaluation summary, 79–80
Reports. *See also* Logs; Records
instrument automation logbook, 192
retrospective Evaluation Summary Report,
97–98

Reports. *See also* Logs; Records
SQAP problems, 116, 118
validation, 57, 62
validation test summary, 69–71, 72
verification, 54–55
Residual material, 153
Restricted access, 11–12
Result logs
in retrospective evaluation package, 80
of legacy system, 96
system owner's validation testing and, 66–68
testing and, 52–53
Retest logs, 88, 90
Retirement
computer system, 31–34, 195–197
system owner's validation role in, 58, 62
Retrospective evaluation package
audit reports and QC reports, 74–75, 78
Evaluation Summary Report of, 97–98
OECD GLP Consensus Document, 86–88
SOPs in, 80, 83–84, 86–88, 92
system and user documents, 91–92
system owner and team roles in, 80–81, 83, 86,
92–94, 96–97
system sponsor and, 79–81, 98–99
testing, 79–83, 94–96
Reviews. *See* Audits/inspections
RFP (request for proposal)
business needs described in, 19–20
for system owner's Validation Plan, 60
retrospective work and, 83–84
suppliers and, 120
system life cycle phases/activities, 15–17
Risk preventative action, 122
ROI (return on investment)
in computers, 3
reasons for validation, 12–13
validation package's effect on, 58–59
*Rules Governing Medicinal Products in the European
Union Vol. IV*, 145

Safety (personnel and product). *See also* SEQ,
217–218
SCADA (supervisory control and data accquisi-
tion), 8–9, 220, 224
SDD (system design description)
as found in engineering SOPs, 45
C.V. Policy's life cycle model and, 134
engineering team's use of, 46–48
in supplier's verification package, 38
supplier's SDLC QA and, 42
system life cycle phases/activities, 16
URS as model for, 24–25
Validation Test Plan and, 63–64
verification in SDLC, 26–27

304 The Survive and Thrive Guide to Computer Validation

SDLC (system development life cycle)
  audit/inspections for, 179
  building and working codes, 25–26
  C.V. Policy's life cycle model and, 134
  documentation of QA, 42
  document development during, 47–48
  MHW GMP Guideline and, 157–159
  system life cycle phases/activities, 15–16
  testing and verification to SDD, 26–27
  URS and SDD in, 25
  validation and, 58, 62, 78
  visibility of components and software and, 23
Security
  definition, 269
  electronic data, 195
  FDA inspection and regulation of e-records,
    149–151
  inclusion in Needs Analysis Report, 18
  inclusion in RFP, 19
  in operations phase of system life cycle, 29–30
  logical, 12
  of system, 2
  quality assurance of, 9, 11–12
Self-Audit Reports. *See also* Audits/inspections,
    42, 48–49
SEQ (safety, efficacy, quality)
  clinical trials and, 201
  GALP laboratory regulations and, 187
  SQAP risk analysis and, 102, 108, 124
Service Level Agreement (SLA), 22
Shutdown of system, 153
Signatures. *See also* e-records; Electronic records
  electronic, 149–152, 163, 255–256, 268, 288–289
  handwritten, 150
Site monitoring. *See* Audits
Software applications
  definition, 269
  design team and verification of, 6
  importance of supplier's verification package,
    55–56
  ladder logic, 8–9
  media storage and retrieval, 119
  QA and audits of, 114–115, 117
Software application system, of operating envi-
    ronment, 6–7
Software application systems, responsibilities of
    owner and team concerning, 34–35
Software development
  code management system and, 45–46
  EDQ Plan and, 211, 213
Software life cycle (definition), 275
Software systems
  acquisition (IEEE Std. 1062-1993), 20, 22–23
  FDA Blue Book inspections and, 153–154
  quality management and assurance of, 20–21

testing and test plans, 52
testing for SDD compliance, 26–27
verification and validation plans, 77–78, 81
Software Verification and Validation Plans, 61–63
SOPs
  as audit and review standards, 169, 173, 176
  e-data integrity and, 203, 209
  electronic records archiving, 196–197
  engineering information included in, 43–45,
    47–48
  FDA Blue Book, 153
  for code and media control, 119, 122
  for OECD GLP legacy system, 87–88, 92
  for Operation Phase Validation, 72–73
  GALP laboratory regulations and, 187–189
  GMP manufacturing systems and, 224–227
  in multiple system environment, 103
  in retrospective evaluation package, 80, 83–84,
    86–88, 92
  in supplier's verification package, 38
  in system owner's validation package, 58, 62
  MHW GMP Guidelines and, 160
  of e-records, 231–232
  quality assurance of, 9–11
  retrospective work and, 80, 83–84, 86–88, 92
  SQAP, 113–115
  supplier management, 120
  supplier's SDLC QA and, 42
Source code, definition, 269
Source data, definition, 280, 287
Source documents, definition, 280, 287
Sponsor. *See* System sponsor
SQAP (Systems Quality Assurance Plan)
  as audit and review standards, 169, 173, 176
  branch testing, 115
  combination testing, 115–117
  configuration management and, 116, 118
  corrective action levels and, 119
  C.V. Policy and, 135–140
  GALP laboratory regulations and, 187–188, 191
  GMP manufacturing systems and, 223–224,
    226, 233
  GOPs of, 113–114
  plan and development of, 104–107
  responsibilites of team, 106–109, 111
  risk management, 122
  signature approval of, 122–123
  system sponsor and, 101–103
  system testing of, 115–117
  system user role in, 110
  training, 121
  verification of qualification, 116
Standard operating procedures. *See* SOPs
Standards. *See also* Regualtions
  EPA 2185 GALP, 184–186, 270–275

Index   305

EU GMP Guide Annex 11, 218–220
FDA 21 CFR Part 11, 230–232
for reviews, audit, or inspections, 169
IEEE Std. 1012-1986, 43–44, 81–82, 61–63
IEEE Std. 1012-1987, 77–78
IEEE Std. 1016.1-1993, 47
IEEE Std. 1016-1987, 47
IEEE Std. 1062-1993, 20, 22–23
IEEE Std. 610.12-1990, 51–52
IEEE Std. 730-1989, 104–105
IEEE Std. 829-1983, 95, 65, 67
IEEE Std. Glossary of Software Engineering
    Terminology, 166–167
ISO 9000-3, 20–21, 39–41, 169
ISO 9000-3:1991, 120–121
ISO 9000 in NAR, 18
SQAP, 111, 113
Standard system model, 133, 138–139
Statement testing, 115
Sterile environment record-keeping, 230–232
Stokes, T., 71, 181
Structural testing, 115–117
Study monitoring systems, 204
Subunit testing, 45
Supplier of system
    purchaser's representative and, 40–42
    Quality Plan and Self-Audit Reports of, 48–49
    representative of, 41–42
    roles in SQAP, 110
    SOPs and control of, 120
    SOPs of SDLC QA and, 42
    verification package and, 37–39
    verification resources and, 39–41
    verification testing and, 49–51
    verification tests and test plans, 51–55
Supplier's Proposal, 20
System documents. *See* Documents
System management logs, 88–91
System owner
    as purchaser's representative, 41
    audit responsibilities, 115
    GALP laboratory regulations and, 186–190
    responsibilities and roles, 15–17
    responsibilities in supplier activities, 120
    responsibilities in system life cycle, 34
    role in C.V. Policy, 127–130, 134–135
    role in inspections and regulations, 171–
        173, 175
    role in IQ and OQ, 27–29
    role in operation phase validation, 71–72
    role in retrospective evaluation, 80–81, 83, 86,
        92–94, 96–97
    role in validation training, 75–76
    role of, 2–4
    roles in SQAP, 102, 104–108, 110, 112

trial sponsor systems and, 203
unannounced FDA inspections and, 168–169
validation package and, 59, 78
validation package of, 57–59, 77–78
Validation Plan of, 60–63, 78
System. *See* Computerized system
System shutdown, 153
Systems (multiple), 102–103
System SOPs. *See* SOPs
System sponsor
    audit perspectives and, 165–168
    budgeting role, 2–4
    clinical research systems and, 199–203
    general role in validation, 1–4
    international regulations and, 143–145
    laboratory systems and, 183–186
    manufacturing system and, 217–219
    responsibilities and roles in system life cycle,
        15–17
    responsibilities in supplier activities, 120
    role in C.V. Policy, 125–129, 134–135, 139–140
    role in Evaluation Summary Report, 79–80
    SQAP and, 101–103, 108, 110–112
    supplier's verification package and, 37–39
    unannounced FDA inspections and, 168–169
    validation package and, 57, 59, 77–78
Systems Quality Assurance Plan. *See* SQAP
System supplier. *See* Supplier of system
System team. *See also* System owner
    as third party site in nonsponsor systems, 203
    components and process of, 3–4
    C.V. Policy and, 133–135
    implementation of Validation Plan by, 57,
        77–78
    representative of, 4, 6
    role in C.V. Policy, 134–136, 138–140
    role in IQ and OQ, 27–29
    SQAP testing responsibilities and, 116
    Transition Summary Report and, 34
System Validation Team, 2. *See also* System team

Tailings accountability, 153
Team. *See* System owner; System team
Testing
    audit/inspection and, 182
    commission, 70–71
    data for, 52–53
    engineering SOPs and, 45
    FDA Blue Book inspections and, 153–154
    GMP manufacturing systems and, 220
    in SDLC, 26–27, 29
    instrument automation logbook and, 192
    retrospective plan and evaluation, 79–83, 94–96
    SQAP, 115–117
    strategy for, 45, 51–52

306 The Survive and Thrive Guide to Computer Validation

system acceptance and, 27–28
validation, 8–9, 63–64, 66–68, 72–75
verification of software, 49–50
Test Log. *See* Result Log
Test Plans
 standard system validation packages and,
  138–139
 supplier's verification package and, 51–52
 validation, 64–65, 69–71, 78
Test scripts, 52–53
 in retrospective evaluation package, 80
 of legacy system, 96
 SQAP testing for GMP systems and, 117
 system owner's validation testing and, 66–68
Tests. *See also specific test name*
 documentation of, 51–55
 in system owner's validation package, 58, 62
 retrospective, 80
Test Summary Report, 54
Timeline of system, 81, 83–85
Traceability testing, 45–46
Training
 audit/inspection and, 182
 in operations phase of system life cycle, 29–30
 in supplier's verification package, 38
 in system owner's validation package, 58,
  62, 72
 management responsibilities, 127
 personnel, 227–228
 preparation for audits/inspections, 232–233
 quality assurance of, 9–10
 validation package and, 75–76
 Validation Plan requirements and SQAP, 121
Training materials
 legacy system use and, 92
 supplier's verification testing and, 51
Transition Plan and Report, 32–34
Trial sponsor systems
 clincial research and, 201–203, 214–215
 general validation package, 204

Unit testing, 26, 45
URS (user requirements specification)
 as model for SDD, 24–25
 contents of, 20
 C.V. Policy's life cycle model and, 134
 document development and control of, 47
 supplier control and, 120
 system life cycle phases/activities, 15–17, 20
 system owner's validation role in, 58, 62
 Validation Test Plan and, 63–64, 139
U.S. Environmental Protection Agency. *See* EPA
User documents. *See* Documents
User manual. *See* Training materials
User Requirements Document, 92

U.S. Food and Drug Administration. *See* FDA
U.S. Pharmaceutical Manufacturers Association
 (PMA), 5. *See also* PMA

Validation
 "worst case" for testing of, 155
 definitions, 1–2, 269
 inclusion in RFP, 19
 in operation phase, 71–72
 lack of retrospective documentation, 91–92
 of VSS, 113
 priority in GMP manufacturing systems,
  217–219
 reasons for, 12–13
 retrospective evaluation package and, 97–98
 risks of, 122
 SEQ risk analysis and, 102, 108
 SQAP tasks and responsibilities, 111–112,
  123–124
 Summary Report, 57, 76–78, 139
Validation Executive Committee
 C.V. Policy and, 128–130, 132, 135–137, 140
Validation package
 budgeting, 58
 GALP laboratory regulations and, 189–190
 general trial sponsor systems, 204
 importance for inspection, 171–172, 177–179
 legacy automation system in, 193–194
 manufacturing system SOPs in, 223–227, 233
 QA and, 75–78
 system owner and team roles in, 57–59, 62,
  71–72, 77–78
Validation Plan
 code and media control, 119, 122
 in commission phase of SDLC, 28–29
 requirements for training, 121
 system owner's, 60–63, 78
Validation testing, 63–64
 of platform system, 8–9
 ongoing QA and QC, 74–75
Validation Test Plan, 64–65, 78
 Test Summary Report and, 69–71, 78
Verification
 by software design team, 6
 SQAP testing qualification and, 116
 testing of software, 49–50
Verification package
 contents of, 38, 41–44
 importance of, 55–56
 system sponsor and, 37–39
 system supplier and, 39–40
 Verification Summary Report and, 54–55
Verification plan
 contents, 44
 of supplier of system, 38, 42–43

Verification Summary Report, contents of, 54–55
Very small system (VSS), validation of, 111, 113

Walk-through review
GALP laboratory regulations and, 186–187
IRT and, 172–176
legacy automation system, 193–194
of GMP manufacturing systems, 221–223,
228–230, 233
QA and, 172–176
WAN. *See* Wide area network
Way Forward Business Plan, 130
GCP, 203
GMP manufacturing systems and, 224
system owner and, 179–180
White box testing, SQAP, 27, 115–117
Wide area network (WAN), 8